SYNOPSIS

This is the first of a proposed series of books that are designed to reveal information that could lead to freedom from suffering and all forms of sickness. It is a practical guide to managing your own health from both a spiritual and physical point of view. It is a distillation of knowledge derived from a lifetime dedication to healing using harmless natural means and remedies. It is aimed at fulfilling a great need for more knowledge of what disease really is, its source and how to overcome it and prevent its manifestation.

The rational nature of Man is the spark of the true light; it is the first step on the upward road.

The power of choice is yours

NATURAL HEALING KNOWLEDGE

Be Educated not Medicated

"Let food be thy medicine and medicine be thy food."

BOOK 1
Recovery, Relief, Health and Longevity
Essential Vital Information

Thomas D'Amico N.D., B.E.
Naturopathic Physician

First edition November 2012

The National Library of Australia Cataloguing-in-Publication entry:

Author:	Thomas D'Amico
Title:	Natural Healing Knowledge: essential knowledge. Book 1/Thomas D'Amico
ISBN:	978-0-9874-4660-2
Subject:	Health
Dewey Number	613

Published by Intertype
A Division of I & E group Pty Ltd
Unit 45, 125 Highbury Road
BURWOOD VIC 3125
Australia
+61 3 9830 6619
contact@intertype.com.au
www.intertype.com.au

CONTENTS:

References:
1. The Natural Healer's Handbook and
2. The Revival of Herbal Wisdom by Thomas D'Amico N.D., B.E.
3. *A Course in Miracles*, published by the Foundation for Inner Peace, Mill Valley, CA 94942, USA

INTRODUCTION
An Awakening from Fear and Deception
Adapted from "The Revival of Herbal Wisdom"

This is an outline of my experience of a process of healing that is still taking place as I write this Introduction. I wish to share my experience regarding the cause and remedy of sickness, hoping that it will shed some light on the subject of healing and bring hope to those in need.

Healing has become a controversial subject, since there are various belief systems and self-promoting vested interests. Why waste your efforts on meaningless arguments that deplete your vitality and lead to nowhere but confusion? True healing requires a willingness to change the mind; deluded minds are not so easily changed. It is the mind that decides whether a given "remedy" will work or not. *The mind makes all decisions that are responsible for the body's condition;* an open clear mind is a great asset!

In early June 2009 I was admitted to hospital as I had become practically lifeless, bed-ridden and physically wasting away. It had been what seemed to be a sudden blow, and I had no energy to help myself in any way; I was losing interest in this world.

There at the hospital, after a period of isolation (I was told that I had a severe and contagious gastro-intestinal infection and the worst case of inflammatory bowel disease ever seen at that hospital), extensive diagnostics involving many CAT scans, x-rays, blood tests and so on, I was informed that I had bowel cancer that had metastasised to the liver. In the current medical belief system such a prognosis would be like a death sentence. I understood that under these circumstances, giving way to fear would be counter productive – cancer does not need to be seen as a death sentence; the seemingly hopeless condition *can* be undone as you allow healing to replace sickness, I thought.

Eventually a major surgical procedure was undertaken but nothing could be done; there were many adhesions and abnormal growths and the tumours could not be removed, and so they sewed me up again and recommended "aggressive" medical treatment to "shrink" the tumours and growths as soon as I gained some strength. The treatment was stopped earlier than planned because I developed severe bowels obstruction and kidney failure.

I was subsequently readmitted to hospital for another major surgical procedure. To cut a long story short, I was eventually sent home and offered palliative care, which I never accepted; I was not expected to live very long. My weight had decreased from about 80 kilos to a skeletal 55 and the cancer was spreading. I experienced constant pain and my energy level was extremely low. My interest in the illusory yet seductive glamour of the world waned as I thought, with ironical amusement that - the masquerade is over. Was the hallucinating - hero of the dream - ready to escape from a world of limitation, suffering and contradiction? Then I saw that immense bright clear Light. This was the turning point.

On the 6th of February 2011 I was facing a determined oncologist who seemed disappointed that I had not chosen his preferred medical treatment and that I was not struck by the terror of death as he repeatedly exclaimed that I didn't realize the "seriousness" of the situation. I just could not take his "death" predictions seriously. I guess that was his way of helping me to "understand". I did not give in to fear nor did I accept the oncology doctor's projection as real, but remained positive and optimistic.

In this game of life you meet messengers of *fear* and messengers of *love*. I realized that the messengers of fear manage this world; they offer you many opportunities for forgiveness; they may appear to know but do they really know what they do? In the dream of pain and suffering that we appear to live in, deluded minds would not see beyond the physical body's experience ending in death, whilst estimating how long you may still be alive in a sick body. If you believed and integrated those kinds of thoughts in your sub-conscious memory, then you would experience that projection. It was just an opinion based on a thought system that I do not choose to accept since it is not in my best interest.

In contrast to the condemning voice, the Messenger of Love explained that:

> As a sovereign being there is no power that
> has ordained your life to be either long-lived or
> short. So, my love, live well in all aspects of
> your life and prosper.

It is now February 8, 2013; I see a troubled world but *is* this reality? How do my thoughts and beliefs influence what I see? I am advised that the world we see is nothing more than a mental construct and sickness is an illusion; time and space are not reality although we believe that they are. Am I completely healed? I know that there is still work to do and much to be shared; let the process of healing continue until it's done, until the mind that sleeps is cleared and unified, all erroneous delusional thinking and mistaken beliefs corrected.

I now accept that true healing involves restoring the mind's integrity. I am willing to allow the undoing of the unconscious guilt, release all fear and realize that every challenge is an opportunity for progress! Healing of the mind may then be reflected in the body and open the way to greater awareness, happiness and joy.

Now I understand that sickness in whatever form it may appear, like cancer for example, is like a shadow that is cast by an idea that obscures the light and that this idea or thought is stored in the sub-conscious mind. You cannot heal cancer by trying to wipe or destroy the shadow but you can make it disappear by removing the idea or belief that is casting the shadow of darkness. Ignorance is another term for darkness. And Light also means knowledge or awareness. Where the Light shines the darkness disappears, so you can choose to be in the Light rather that darkness.

It is your choice whether you listen to the Voice for truth or that other voice, which tells you things that are not in your best interest and which lead to confusion and suffering. The key lies in the belief system that has been accepted as reality in your sub-conscious mind. Accept then the reality of peace, healing, happiness and abundance as the eternal attributes of the real you and reject suffering, pain and death which are projections from the mind that sleeps and dreams of disaster.

Believe it or not:
"All forms of sickness, even unto death, are physical expressions of the fear of awakening."
From: *A Course in Miracles*, published by The Inner Peace Foundation, USA.

∗∗∗

THE CRITICAL FACTOR

It may be difficult or even impossible for individuals to accept that everything that appears to happen in the physical world, which includes your body, is a projection of thoughts and beliefs in the subconscious mind. It is an error to think that the mind resides in the body. The body is an idea within the mind that believes in separation and this thought is projected as an outward appearance.

It would appear as if medicines and therapies do have a purpose in this world, to make the body better. Therapies aim to heal the body and you may experience an improvement, deterioration or no measurable effect, depending on complex individual issues. When symptoms vanish and you feel better, you may think that you have been cured, at least temporarily. However, unless the sub-conscious belief system is changed the sickness will be projected again at a different time, maybe in a different form, because there has been no change in the mind's choice of belief system. The same mental program is still in place. The appearance of sickness is then likely to be reactivated especially when the patient experiences prolonged stressful situations.

Under stressful circumstances the sympathetic part of the autonomic nervous system is activated, the cells shut down and go into the "fight-or-flight" protection mode. Your cells are then closed and unable to receive sufficient oxygen and essential nutrients or release waste products.

Stress is not caused by external circumstances. In his research at Stanford University, Dr. Bruce Lipton Ph. D., renowned cellular biologist and author of The Biology of Belief, was able to prove in the laboratory, that it is wrong beliefs [or wrong perception] which reside in our subconscious mind, that create stress in our autonomic nervous system. These wrong beliefs cause us to interpret our circumstances as stressful, even when they aren't.

According to Dr. Lipton, an authority on bridging science and the spirit, the difference between the closed cell and a cell that is open (i.e., in "growth mode") is that the cell that's in growth mode is impervious to disease.

When a cell goes into lock down, fight-or-flight mode, that cell is not getting oxygen, not absorbing nutrients, not properly eliminating waste products, and not functioning the way it normally should. If the cell remains in that state for a short period of time, the effects are inconsequential.

That's why a small amount of stress in life rarely leads to health problems. But if the cell stays in the closed, fight-or-flight mode for an extended period of time, it becomes a sick cell. The main reason for this is because of the lack of oxygen. When you choose to remain in a stressful situation or a stressed-out state of mind, that's equivalent to suffocating your body and depriving it of the element that it needs most to survive[1].

As it is simply expressed in The One Minute Cure: "If stress rules your life, your cells will be sick and remain sick because they're frequently closed and unable to receive or absorb any remedy you provide."

Fear, guilt, hatred, resentment and anger are the cause of all human ailments and pain, which thrive when Love is withheld.

✳✳✳

---

[1] From The One Minute Cure, The Secret of Healing Virtually All Diseases, by Madison Cavanaugh, 2008.

Module 1.
JOURNEY TO RECOVERY

Vital Information for Cancer Patients

PART 1. THE KEY – A Summary

Cancer is like a fungus, which can grow and spread quickly if not kept under control, especially when there's infected damaged tissue that doesn't seem to heal. Cancer tumours are composed of fungal tissue called *Ergosterol.* As well as killing the cancer and prevent it from spreading, it is important to support the immune system and regenerate the body to repair damage caused by the cancer and the effects of chemical drugs, chemotherapy and radiation. High fever kills cancer cells and disease cells cannot tolerate a high level of oxygenation.

Consider these in consultation with a competent and caring physician:
- **Restore your purpose in life and deal with unresolved emotional issues** – realize that there's nothing to gain from being sick. Feelings of guilt, despair and hopelessness can suppress the activity of the immune system. Such feelings arise from delusional thinking – these are illusions held in the sub-conscious mind that must be corrected for healing to occur.

- Research shows that the Immune System needs 9 1/2 hours of sleep in *total* darkness to recharge completely – avoid caffeine.

- Note and choose the specific remedies, which are indicated for the form of cancer being treated. Work out a daily program that suits you.

- Boost Immune System and prevent its deterioration. Consider taking Beta 1.3 & 1.6 Glucan, herbal remedies, wild herbs and fresh organic whole foods that boost immunity and kill cancer cells without harming normal cells.

Alkalise the body to optimal pH of 8 to encourage an oxygen-rich environment – e.g. Consider Sodium Bicarbonate, Caesium chloride, Green and White tea, Yerba Mate tea, Barley Grass, Chlorophyll and Fresh Green Herbs, Fruit and

Vegetables, which are high in Salvestrols[2]. **The Sodium-Bicarbonate-Molasses treatment has been used successfully in prostate and bone cancer.**

- Eliminate detrimental fungus, moulds and parasites. Herbal combinations can be safe and very effective in eliminating these infections and prevent the cancer from spreading.

- Take Digestive Enzymes to dissolve the protein coating that protects the cancer cells thus inhibiting their destruction.

- Take foods and remedies to restore the damage caused by the cancer and conventional medical treatment (e.g. take Glutathione[3] restoring foods and herbs together with Green Super Foods).

- Prevent vascularization of tumours (Angiogenesis)[4].

- Dr Johanna Budwig's flaxseed oil and sulphur-based protein therapy has helped to cure cancer, even terminal cancer. This consists in taking 3-4 tablespoons flaxseed oil blended with ½ cup low-fat quark once daily. **Avoid** canola oil, Olestra, Margarine and processed foods containing harmful fats and oils, canned tomatoes, carcinogenic chemicals and food additives[5].

---

[2] **Salvestrols** are a new class of natural anti-cancer chemicals found in certain dietary plants and fruits. Salvestrols have the extraordinary ability to recognize cancer cells, embed themselves in them and destroy them. Refer to page 392 The Revival of Herbal Wisdom, for more details.

[3] **Glutathione** has been called "The Mother of all Antioxidants".
[4] Angiogenesis inhibiting remedies: Watercress, Turmeric, Ashwagandha, Chinese red sage root and Shark's cartilage.
[5] Industrially prepared packaged foods may contain chemicals (such as MSG) that make the cancer grow faster, making it incurable. Also avoid smoked foods, fried foods and preserved meats and synthetic vitamins, colouring and additives. There are more than 3000 food additives and some of them are known carcinogens. Additives that may be safe individually may form harmful compounds in certain combinations. Avoid Canola Oil as this releases toxic carcinogenic fumes when heated.

PART 2. HEALING THE MIND

Exercise your mind's power to choose what is in your best interest. You can choose wellness instead of sickness; choose forgiveness instead of judgment and choose love rather than fear for yourself and others. You need to face your emotional issues reasonably and in a space of stillness, non-judgment and forgiveness.

You need to restore the awareness of **your purpose** for 'being here'. Your mind *must* have a purpose to keep the body alive and well! You may think that you no longer have a purpose or that you do not know what your purpose is. Rest assured that there is a purpose for appearing here in a body; there is nothing to gain by being sick. Identify yourself with your strength and not your weakness!

- Think beyond the body – everyone is you appearing in a different body. The question is: who is that "you" – that is your true identity?
- Do not give into fear or guilt that diminish you and enslave you.
- There is no need for sacrifice but be willing to change your perception.
- Let your purpose be happiness, free from all suffering and pain.
- Free your mind from judgment and false beliefs.
- The Truth will indeed set you free.

PART 3. HARMFUL SUBSTANCES

Substances that accelerate cancer growth making the cancer incurable
- Monosodium Glutamate (MSG) and its derivatives, used in many processed foods as a "flavour enhancer".
- Aspartame.
- Tobacco smoking.
- Talcum powder.
- Formaldehyde – when the Methanol content of Aspartame enters the body, it is converted to

Formaldehyde. Other sources are: cigarette smoke, Cleansers, Plastic Furniture, Nail Polish, Pressed wood, New Carpet etc.
- Detrimental yeasts and moulds.
- Parasites.
- Preserved or smoked meats and meat injected with Growth Hormones.
- Foods fried in vegetable oils, and barbequed meats.
- Micro waved foods.

Foods that cause inflammation.
- Refined sugar (use Stevia, Xylitol or coconut sugar).
- Table salt (use Celtic sea salt or Himalayan salt).
- Red meat, smoked meat and smoked fish, barbequed meat.
- Chlorinated water.
- Alcohol.
- Fast foods.
- Foods fried in vegetable oil.
- Margarine.
- Coffee.
- Black tea.
- Soft drinks.
- Potato chips.
- Peanuts and peanut butter.
- Pasteurized and homogenized cows milk. Ice cream. Cheddar cheese.
- Microwave cooked/heated foods.
- Reconstituted, canned, bottled or frozen juices.

PART 4. ELIMINATION AND RESTORATION

* SPECIFICS
Researchers have revealed certain specific substances for the type of cancer.
These substances together with the cause of the cancer are given on The Natural Healer's Handbook as well as The Revival of Herbal Wisdom.
Ideally a specific program would need to be arranged for individual needs and this program revised as required.

* REMEDIES TO ELIMINATE CANCER
Substances that destroy cancer without harming normal cells

Obviously it would not be practical to take <u>all</u> of these remedies every day so a program with guidelines to include these remedies into your protocol would be advised.

- Digestive enzymes – to dissolve the protective protein coat around cancer cells.
- Dr Johanna Budwig's protocol[6] of combining and blending about two-thirds of a cup of organic low fat **cottage cheese** or **quark** with one-third cup of **flaxseed oil**. It must be blended - stirring isn't good enough for it to be effective in destroying cancer cells[7]. This is taken as a meal once daily; you can add one heaped tablespoon of **freshly ground flaxseeds**, fruit, almonds or walnuts to the mixture if you wish. **This must be taken well away from Hydrogen Peroxide as explained in The Revival of Herbal Wisdom, page 398 "Oxygen Therapy". Hemp seeds oil can be used instead of the Flaxseed oil**
- Hydrogen peroxide 35% food grade procedure – diluted as directed by physician. This must not be taken together with fats such as in the Budwig's diet as this would form lipid peroxides and damage stomach lining.
- Laetrile – Vitamin B17 – highest source is Apricot Kernels.
- Salvestrols – contained in **organic produce** (fruits and vegetables) and organic or wild crafted herbs.
- Lemon Juice added to purified water.
- Chlorophyll added to drinking water.
- Sodium bicarbonate – taken half hour before meals to make the body more alkaline.

---

[6] Researchers in Germany (Budwig and others) found that anaerobic that spawns the proliferation of cancer is caused by a lack of sufficient Omega-3 and Omega-6 essential fatty acids in the diet as well as the overconsumption of modern processed foods containing unhealthy forms of fats and oils.

[7] In his book (How to Cure Almost any Cancer at Home for $5.15 a day) Bill Anderson writes that, based on experience, this simple food combination has a 90% success rate at curing cancer – especially terminal cancer.

- Kombu seaweed – contains *fucoidan*, which destroys cancer and prevents radiation damage.
- **Herbal remedies** – Anti-fungal/Mould elimination/Parasites elimination/Anti-tumour & Anti-cancer herbal remedies.

*REMEDIES FOR RESTORATION[8]

ORGANIC RAW FOODS – refer to the Revival of Herbal Wisdom Part 4, Natural Cancer Elimination Strategies
- Asparagus
- Chia seeds
- Broccoli and Tomato combination
- Mung-bean sprouts
- Almonds – soaked overnight
- Pecans, Walnuts
- Green tea, White tea, Tulsi tea, Yerba Santa tea.
- Wild Herbs are Nature's Extraordinary Healers. Such herbs as: Dandelion, Herb Robert, Fat Hen, Purslane, Parsley, Fennel, Wild Lettuce, Sheep Sorrel, Nasturtium, Mint etc.
- Apricots and apricot kernels (B17), Papaya, Radishes, Turnips, Watercress, Kiwi fruit, pineapple, apples – eat the core as well (seeds contain Laetrile -vitamin B17).
- Organic Juices such as: Pomegranate, Mangosteen, Goji berry puree, Blueberries, Acai Berries and Sea Buckthorn (oil and fruit).

Adopt an Alkaline Forming Diet
Refer to The Natural Healer's Handbook
- Sodium Bicarbonate taken in water half-hour before meals or as directed by your physician.
- Chlorophyll and foods rich in chlorophyll such as Chlorella.

---

[8] The appropriate herbal remedies will be offered to the patient following a professional consultation.

15

- Have a diet consisting of 80% alkaline forming and 20% acid forming foods. Fruit, vegetables and millet are alkaline forming; meat, eggs, legumes and grains are acid forming.
- Drink natural spring water or purified water with a ph of about 8. Avoid chlorinated/fluoridated tap water.
- Avoid micro-waving foods and drinks.
- Avoid highly acidifying foods and beverages such as: Coffee, Refined sugar, fried foods, Refined Carbohydrates, Foods with added sugar, Alcohol, Soft drinks.
- Eat simply; do not mix too many types of foods at the same meal.
- Do not hurry meals, sit down, relax and enjoy!

Hippocrates, known as the Father of Modern Medicine wrote, "Let your food be your medicine and your medicine be your food". Open minded physicians are more and more speaking out in favor of Nature's marvelous healers; it is the Revival of Herbal Wisdom.

Organic unprocessed foods can heal you in ways drugs never can. It is nature's way to repair, restore and rejuvenate; they heal your body without dangerous side effects.

Peace, Health and Happiness to All!

PART 5. HERBAL FORMULAE

Because of legal restrictions these remedies will generally be considered and offered to individuals following a diagnosis by a competent and suitably qualified physician.

Herbal combinations 1 to 4 have been developed to assist the body in the elimination of abnormal growths and detrimental organisms such as fungi and parasites. Combinations 6 to 10 would assist with the restoration of the organism.

1. Anti-Fungal Herbs

Detrimental Fungi (such as Candida Albicans in its mutated form) can cause allergies and may be responsible for infections such as Tinea and many other ailments including, headaches, depression, lack of vitality and digestive problems. These organisms are nourished largely by sugars.

Cancer Patients practically always show signs of heavy parasitic infestation, as well as the open ileo-caecal valve syndrome.

Indications: Candida Albicans overload and detrimental Yeast Infections, Mould elimination, Bloating, Joints Pain, Low Energy level, Thrush, Tinea.

Remedies selected:
- *Cinnamon*
- *Garlic*
- *Horsetail*
- *Horseradish*
- *Myrrh*
- *Neem leaf*
- *Nigella Sativa seeds*
- *Pau D'Arco*
- *Mountain pepper (Tasmannia lanceolata)*
- *Vitamin C (ascorbic acid)*
- *Zinc oxide*

NOTE: When the Candida organisms die, yeast toxins are rapidly released into the blood stream, usually in excess of the liver's capacity. A "die off" reaction is felt, where there is a transient worsening of symptoms. Herbs that support liver and kidney function will reduce this tendency.

2. Parasites Elimination Herbs

Indications: Parasites may be transmitted to humans through insect bites, drinking contaminated water, and eating undercooked meat and fish. Raw fruits and vegetables can harbour parasites. Parasites can get into the body by putting unwashed hands into the mouth after they have been in contact with something that contains parasites. Close contact with companion pets and other animals is another way of acquiring parasites. The size of parasites can range from microscopic amoebas to worms that can grow a metre or more in length.

Remedies Selected:
- *Barberry*
- *Black walnut green hull*
- *Bistort root*
- *Cloves*
- *Garlic*
- *White horehound*
- *Neem leaf*
- *Wormwood*
- *MSM*
- *Ascorbic acid*

3. Mould Elimination Herbs

Indications: Parasites, Detrimental yeasts and Mould infestation, Flatulence and intestinal cramps.

Remedies Selected:
- *Cassia Cinnamon*
- *Coriander*
- *Citrus rind*
- *Cumin*
- *Black cumin*
- *Nigella*

Nutmeg
Peppermint
Star anise
Schizandra
Ascorbic acid

4. Anti-Tumour Herbs

Indications: Liver toxicity, Tumours and Growths, Cancer, Low Immunity and Inflammations.

Remedies Selected:
- *Astragalus root*
- *Black fungus*
- *Fo-Ti*
- *Herb Robert*
- *Cat's claw*
- *Dan Shen*
- *Turmeric*
- *Ginger*
- *Nigella sativa*
- *Ginkgo biloba*
- *Moringa oleifera*

By far, the most powerful antioxidants are those produced within the body – Glutathione peroxidase, Catalase and Superoxide Dismutase[9]. The following herbal combinations (5 to 10) have been developed in recent times and are designed to help the body stimulate production and increase activity of these endogenous Antioxidant Enzymes.

5. Green Super-Foods Combination.

Indications: Exposure to Radioactivity, Inflammations, Colitis, Arthritis, Cancer, Low Immunity and Toxic Overload.

Remedies Selected:
- *Spirulina*
- *Chlorella*

---

[9] **Selenium** is part of the Glutathione molecule. Australian soils are generally Selenium deficient, so that Selenium rich foods or supplements may be necessary.

- *Barley grass*
- *Moringa oleifera*
- *Ginger*

6. Life Extension Herbs

Indications: Premature Aging, Low Energy Level, Chronic disease, Adrenal Exhaustion, Poor Libido and Low Immunity.

Remedies Selected:
- *Astragalus Root*
- *Panax Ginseng*
- *Grape Seeds and Grape skins powder,*
- *Green tea*
- *Terminalia chebula*
- *Amla and*
- *Silica*
- *Goji Berry*
- *Privet Berry*
- *Rhodiola Rosea*
- *Withania (Ashwagandha)*
- *MSM (Dimethyl- sulfonyl-methane*
- *Vitamin C with Bioflavonoids*

7. Super Herbal Antioxidants

Indications: Stress, Chronic Diseases, Chronic Fatigue Syndrome, Premature Aging, Weakness and Free Radicals toxic overload.

Remedies Selected:
- *Ashwagandha*   *Cacao (raw unprocessed)*
- *Grape seeds powder*   *Acai berry*
- *Grape skin powder*   *Fo-Ti*
- *Green tea*   *Reishi mushrooms*

8. Protection Glutathione Herbs

Glutathione is a potent anti-oxidant. It binds to toxin in the liver, the body's primary cleansing organ, and allow them to be flushed efficiently. A deficiency in Glutathione plays a major role in premature aging, low sperm count, liver and heart disease, diabetes and cancer.

Indications: Toxic overload (chemicals, drugs, pesticides and heavy metals), Glutathione depletion, premature aging, liver and heart disease, diabetes, low immunity, arthritis and cancer.

Remedies Selected:

- *Ashwagandha*   *Moringa*
- *Curcumin*   *Satavari*
- *Cardamom*   *Piperine*
- *Cinnamon*   *Terminalia chebula*
- *Ginger*

Food Sources of Glutathione:

Raw fruit and vegetables: Asparagus (leading source of Glutathione), Onion, Garlic, Globe artichoke, Tomato, Spinach, Broccoli, Kale, Brussels sprouts, Cauliflower, Avocado, Lemon and Grapefruit. Walnuts, Brazil nuts, raw eggs, freshly prepared rare or raw meat, raw unpasteurised non-homogenised milk, yoghurt and wheat germ.

Undenatured (non-heated) cold processed whey protein is one of the natural foods known to selectively deplete cancer cells of their glutathione, thus making them more susceptible to such cancer treatments as radiation and chemotherapy.

9. Vigour SOD & Catalase Herbs

Superoxide Dismutase (SOD) is an endogenous enzyme, antioxidant and anti-inflammatory agent with anti-aging and cancer preventative properties.

Indications: Chronic Inflammation, Crohn's Disease, Inflammatory Bowel Disease, Corneal ulcers, Burns and Injuries, Exposure to smoke and Radiation[10], Cancer, Liver disease, Heart weakness, Arthritis and Prostate problems.

Remedies Selected:
- *Ashwagandha*   *Milk Thistle*
- *Brahmi*   *Green tea*
- *Ginkgo biloba*   *Parsley*
- *Amla*
- *Korean Ginseng*

10. Vigour and Zest

Indications: Adaptogen Tonic, Anti-cancer, Stress and Memory loss.

Remedies Selected:
- *Ashwagandha*   *Amla*
- *Tulsi*   *Mint*
- *Satavari*   *Zest (citrus rind)*

---

[10] **Exposure to radiation** causes a cascade of free radicals that wreak havoc on the body. Radiation also decimates the body's supply of glutathione, which allows free radicals to run rampant through our body's tissues and organs. Though there might be some kind of hormesis effect with an up-tick of glutathione body defences, it is vital to understand that glutathione levels cannot be sustained without all the precursors being supplied—namely selenium, magnesium and sulphur.

Medical Imaging Radiation

The latest published data on radiation exposure suggests that **roughly 25,000 Americans develop cancer every year as a result of medical radiation exposure**, and many more experience DNA damage that could eventually lead to the development of cancer and other health problems in the long term.

Many people undergo computed tomography (CT), positron emission tomography (PET), magnetic resonance imaging (MRI), and X-ray scans for medical purposes, thinking that by doing so, they are keeping up with the latest technologies in advanced medical care. But each time medical patients get one of these scans, their bodies sustain varying levels of ionizing radiation, the negative effects of which can take years to manifest as they build up cumulatively over time.

CT scans, which are a relatively modern medical imaging technology, are particularly problematic as they emit far higher doses of radiation than traditional x-rays do. Based on the figures, a single CT scan can blast up to 500 times the amount of radiation released by a single x-ray, an astounding level when considering how gratuitously CT scans are administered within the medical profession today.

In a new study recently published in the *Journal of the American Medical Association* (JAMA), it is reported that the use of all medical imaging scans, including CT scans, has risen dramatically between 1996 and 2010. The use of CT scans in particular, more than tripled during this time, which is in large part responsible for doubling the proportion of patients now receiving what is considered to be "high" or "very high" radiation doses on a regular basis.

∗∗∗

Module 2
PAIN RELIEF

WHAT HEALS & WHAT KILLS?
Drugless Natural Alternative

25

1. PHARMACEUTICAL DRUGS EFFECTS

Medications intended to decrease pain can actually end up increasing the risk for heart attack, stroke and liver disease, as well as gastrointestinal, kidney and blood pressure problems. These medicines should not be taken for lengthy periods of time.

Non Steroidal Anti-Inflammatory Drugs

Advil, Aleve, Motrin, ibuprofen and naproxen are all types of NSAIDs (non-steroidal, anti-inflammatory drugs) that reduce pain, inflammation and fever. The short-term pain relief these OTCs provide comes with several high prices:

> * Gastrointestinal bleeding.
> * Stomach ulcers.
> * Fluid retention and possible oedema.
> * Increased blood pressure.
> * Kidney failure.
> * Liver failure.

According to several medical studies, including a recent report published in *BMJ* (formerly the *British Medical Journal*), NSAIDs also increase your risk of heart attack and stroke. Scientists from the University of Bern in Switzerland analyzed data from 31 clinical trials that consisted of over 116,000 patients. The investigation revealed that stroke victims had been taking a normal recommended dose (400-600 mg) of ibuprofen 3 or 4 times daily.

The Dangers of Acetaminophen

Acetaminophen is the leading ingredient in the popular pain medication, Tylenol. Twenty-eight billion doses of acetaminophen are purchased every year in the United

States alone! Take a look at the consequences of those 28 billion doses:

* 26,000 hospitalizations
* 500 deaths
* 41,000 calls to poison control centres

According to the FDA, Tylenol has replaced viral hepatitis as the **leading cause of acute liver failure**. Unfortunately, the liver starts to deteriorate long before any symptoms manifest.

Aspirin Side Effects

Research has found that regular use of the salicylate drug aspirin deteriorates the intestinal lining, causing severe bleeding, colitis, intestinal perforation, infections and in some cases, even death. Aspirin may be able to alleviate pain, but it also depletes the body of essential minerals and nutrients, damaging vital organs and exacerbating heart conditions. Research indicates that regular use of aspirin is linked to heart attacks and strokes.

Gastroenterologist Dr. Neena S. Abraham reported on the harmful effects of aspirin in a 2010 *New York Times* article:

"It is important to remember that all NSAIDs, including over-the-counter aspirin, have the potential to damage the tissue of the gastrointestinal tract. Damage can occur anywhere, from mouth to anus ... Aspirin is not a nutritional supplement—it is a medication with real risks and side-effects."

Aspirin may also accelerate the process of Joints destruction by chondroclasts.

2. THE NATURAL ALTERNATIVE

You may choose natural alternatives to pharmaceutical drugs, it is up to you and no one should be forced or coerced to choose against their own will. However the choice of remedy requires that you be properly informed and loose your fear of not conforming to a conventional protocol. Not many people are prepared to go against rigidly held beliefs and ideas that are popular in the world of mainstream medicine.

These are safe natural remedies to relieve pain and inflammation:

- **Proteolytic Enzymes (Proteases)**

Proteolytic Enzymes are enzymes that break down proteins. Research indicates these enzymes work throughout your entire body to help it fight inflammation... dissolve scar tissue... cleanse and thin the blood... plus even boost cardiovascular, respiratory and immune function.

Proteolytic enzymes are the final line of defence against disease, illnesses, pain and everything else that happens inside your body.
And unfortunately with the nutrient-deficient food we're eating today, the vast majority of adults today have dangerously low levels of these enzymes!

Dietary Sources of Proteolytic Enzymes: Natto, Miso, Kiwi Fruit, Papaya, Pineapple, Sauerkraut, Kefir and Ginger. Heat (cooking and baking) and processing destroys these enzymes.

- **Herbs and Nutrients**

There are herbs that have been used for thousands of years and lately science has confirmed what was already known about their ability to relieve pain and inflammation.

- Boswellia
- Turmeric
- Ginger
- Devil's Claw
- Citrus Bioflavonoids
- Noni Fruit
- Mojave Yucca (root)
- Chaparral
- Cloves
- Black Cohosh
- White Willow Bark

- **L-Glutathione** *(refer to page 32)*

- **L-Glutamine**

- **Whey Protein (cold processed)**

- **MSM (Methylsulfonylmethane)**

- **Spirulina**

3. HERBAL COMBINATIONS
These herbal mixtures have been developed over the years to relieve pain and restore damaged tissue.

* Anti-Inflammatory Formula

Indications: Inflammatory diseases, Rheumatoid Arthritis, Osteo-Arthritis, Inflammatory Bowel Disease, Bursitis, Irritable Bowels Syndrome, Crohn's Disease and Ulcerative Colitis.

Remedies Selected:
- *Baical skullcap*   *Turmeric*
- *Boswellia serrata*   *Ginger*
- *Buplerum*   *Piperine*
- *Curcumin*

* IBS Soothing Herbs
Powder or Capsules

This combines alkalising minerals and herbs that will soothe Irritable Bowels, help in the repair of damaged mucous membrane and remove excess acidity from the tissue.

Indications: Irritable bowels syndrome, Acid Reflux, Hiatus Hernia, Inflammatory bowels disease, Peptic Ulcer and digestion problems.

Remedies Selected:

1. Calcium carbonate
2. Magnesium carbonate
3. Sodium bicarbonate
4. Peppermint
5. Citric acid
6. Liquorice root
7. White willow bark
8. Slippery elm bark

9. Turmeric
10. Bay leaf
11. Fennel seed
12. Guar gum
13. Glutamine
14. Xylitol or Stevia
15. Asafoetida
16. Cardamom pods

Dosage:

The loose powder is recommended for fast relief when there is acute abdominal pain: half to one teaspoon in water mixed thoroughly and taken away from food or when there's abdominal distress or pain**. In severe cases and where there is constant pain repeat in 15 minutes then half hour until pain is abated.**

* Headaches and Migraines Herbs

Indications: Migraine Headaches, Headaches, Stress and Adrenal Exhaustion.

Remedies Selected:
- *Bay leaves*
- *Feverfew*
- *Ginger*
- *Ginkgo biloba*
- *Peppermint*
- *Passionflower*
- *Rhodiola rosea*

* Joints & Muscle Formula

Indications: Joints pain and Inflammation, Muscle and tendons pain and Inflammation, Fibromyalgia.

Remedies Selected:
- *Boswellia serrata*
- *Curcumin*
- *Piperine*
- *Glucosamine*
- *Celery seeds*
- *Bovine collagen*
- *MSM*
- *Vitamin C*

* Protection Glutathione Herbs

Glutathione is a potent anti-oxidant. It binds to toxin in the liver, the body's primary cleansing organ, and allow them to be flushed efficiently. A deficiency in Glutathione plays a major role in premature aging, low sperm count, liver and heart disease, diabetes and cancer. The following formula is not a Glutathione supplement; the herbs within are known to stimulate the production of endogenous Glutathione.

Indications: Toxic overload (chemicals, drugs, pesticides and heavy metals), Glutathione depletion, premature aging, liver and heart disease, diabetes, low immunity, arthritis and cancer.

Remedies Selected:
- *Ashwagandha*   *Moringa*
- *Curcumin*   *Satavari*
- *Cardamom*   *Piperine*
- *Cinnamon*   *Terminalia chebula*
- *Ginger*

Food Sources of Glutathione:

Raw fruit and vegetables: Asparagus (leading source of Glutathione), Onion, Garlic, Globe artichoke, Tomato, Spinach, Broccoli, Kale, Brussels sprouts, Cauliflower, Avocado, Lemon and Grapefruit. Walnuts, Brazil nuts, raw eggs, freshly prepared rare or raw meat, raw unpasteurised non-homogenised milk, yoghurt and wheat germ.

Undenatured (non-heated) cold processed whey protein is one of the natural foods known to selectively deplete cancer cells of their glutathione, thus making them more susceptible to such cancer treatments as radiation and chemotherapy.

4. LIVER PAIN RELIEF

Where there is pain due to liver toxic overload, Castor Oil fomentations are a quick and simple way to relieve pain in the liver due to congestion. The castor oil will penetrate deeply into the skin to dissolve growths and relieve morbid encumbrances.

Procedure:

- Fill two vessels with water one with hot water and the other with normal cool water.

- Gently spread and rub the Castor Oil all over the skin above the liver area.

- Use two small towels dipping and soaking them, one in each vessel.

- Place the towels alternately over the area with the castor oil.

- Do 4 minutes hot and 1 minute cold. Repeat this for about 20 minutes, 3 times daily or more if you wish.

- Finish with the cold application

Module 3
LIFE EXTENSION

Inhibiting the Aging Process

1. SIGNS OF PREMATURE AGING

The signs of aging includes not only wrinkles, but memory loss, decreased brain function and increasing risk of chronic diseases such as chronic fatigue syndrome, heart disease, osteoporosis and cancer. Many studies have documented a link between a truly healthy diet and the prevention of age-related or chronic diseases.

2. AGENTS THAT CAUSE DEGENERATION AND PREMATURE AGING

- Mental rigidity, Fear, Worry, Stress and Trauma
- Over-consumption of Alcohol
- Poor nutrition
- **Overeating:** eating excessively large meals means that your digestive system struggles to process and assimilate. This creates an accumulation of undigested material and toxic waste products that can cause premature aging and metabolic disorders such as Diabetes.
- **Acid Waste Build-Up** – The typical western diet is acid-forming. Acid forming foods such as meat and potatoes, fried foods, coffee, soft drinks, sucrose and other sugars build up acidic waste products in the body. We need about 25 % acid forming and 75% alkaline forming foods. Stress and worry can also form acidic deposits in the body.
- Aflatoxin Moulds
- Exposure to toxic chemicals and heavy metals
- Excessive exposure to the sun
- Insufficient exposure to sunlight
- Tobacco smoking - produces carbon monoxide *(Hemoglobin's oxygen-binding capacity is decreased in the presence of carbon monoxide because both gases compete for the same binding sites on hemoglobin, carbon monoxide binding preferentially in place of oxygen.)*
- Artificial sweeteners
- Enzymes inhibitors
- Aluminium cookware
- Synthetic chemicals in the air, food, **water** and other beverages.

3. ANTI AGING LIFESTYLE

We live in a world where for every experience or effect that is manifested there is an underlying cause. The choosing of foods that are Anti-inflammatory and rich in Anti-oxidants and enzymes but free from enzyme inhibitors is recommended. Foods that are known to cause Inflammation and undermine your immune system are a sign that your body is reacting to these foods and thus they should be minimized or avoided where possible. Lifestyle should be adjusted to prevent premature aging and disease.

Inflammation causes us to age. Scientists now believe that rampant chronic inflammation can encourage diseases like cancer, heart disease, arthritis, Alzheimer's, diabetes and lupus as well as allergies.

Steps to eliminating inflammation and premature aging:

- **Proper hydration**: dehydration causes an inflammatory response; it makes you feel tired, confused and fearful. Use purified or spring water but avoid drinking tap water that has been contaminated with chlorine, sodium fluoride, aluminium and many other added chemicals.

- **Nutrition:** Avoid stale foods. The key here is to eat and drink foods that do not cause inflammation that are high in enzyme activity and rich in Antioxidants. This means that you would need to eat a certain amount of fresh raw food daily since heat and processing destroys required antioxidants and enzymes in foods.

- **Maintain a healthy weight**: decrease intake of sugars, hydrogenated vegetable oils, fast foods, processed foods, fatty red meat, fried foods and starches. Choose whole foods, especially anti-inflammatory variety such as lean proteins, fruit and vegetables (preferably organically grown). The fatty tissues of the body secrete hormones that regulate the immune system and inflammation, but in the case of an overweight individual this can become out of control. Three of the hormones that play a role in metabolism are *leptin* (involved in appetite control)*, resistin* (increases insulin resistance) *and adiponectin* (lowers the blood sugar by making your body more insulin sensitive). Have Chia seeds in your diet.

- **Get adequate and better quality sleep**: 7 to 9 ½ hours of sleep in complete darkness is essential for optimum health; getting a good night sleep is essential for controlling inflammation. Sleep deprivation can interfere with the way we function mentally and physically. Quality of sleep is one of the essential elements for the restoration of the body. Requirements differ for each individual, but, if you find that during the day you feel irritable, are snappy, get giddy spells and that your cognitive abilities like memory, attention span and concentration are impaired, then, you may be suffering from the cumulative effect of inadequate level of sleep.

- **Relaxation and stress reduction**: each day, find time to sit down or lie down and relax and call upon your true inner strength to guide you, focus on your breathing and be willing for the clutter in your mind to be cleared; stay focused on the most important tasks in your life.

- **Exercise regularly**: aim for 15-20 minutes doing something you like to do, 5 times a week. Swinging the arms is good for the heart and longevity.

- **Nature walks:** The causes of stress are things that our sub-conscious mind perceives as threats. In response to the "real" or imagined stress factors, the brain reacts by directing the secretion of "stress hormones" that produce toxic substances, which are dumped into the bloodstream. This brings about conditions such as: rise in blood pressure, palpitations, anger, fear, worry or aggression. It may be necessary to take time off and walk away from your stressful environment at work or home and do something that you enjoy. Spend time walking and admiring nature's beautiful handiwork, smell the roses, listen to the birds and breath-in the life-giving prana that is there all around you, and it's free!

4. ANTI AGING HERBS

Nature provides many wonderful remedies that help prevent premature aging and restore the life force or lowered vitality. We don't yet understand how they work. Consider the following remedies:

- **Withania** *(Ashwagandha or Indian ginseng)***:** Studies have shown this herb to have many health benefits including: anti-oxidant activity, ability to support a healthy immune system, help the body to adapt to stress as well as anti-aging effects. Scientific studies have indicated that Ashwagandha restores the *Telomeres.* A Telomere is a region of repetitive DNA at the end of a chromosome, which protects the chromosome from degeneration. Many age-related diseases are linked to shortened Telomeres.

- **Acai berry:** A potent antioxidant, which scavenges errand Free Radicals that cause cellular damage and premature aging. It contains Resveratrol, Oligomeric Proantocyanidins (OPCs) and Epicatechin. It has been found to stimulate the death of Leukaemia cells.

- **American ginseng - Key Actions:** Adaptogen, Hypotensive, Tonic (brain, heart and nervous system), Anti-aging, Aphrodisiac, Digestive and Anti-inflammatory

- **Amla fruit - Key Actions:** Adaptogen, Antioxidant, Antipyretic (Anti-inflammatory), Digestive, Astringent, Laxative, Ophthalmic, Carminative, Aphrodisiac and Diuretic.

- **Astragalus root - Key Actions:** Adaptogen, Cardio tonic, Diuretic, Immune stimulating, Anti microbial and Anti viral. Astragalus scavenges free radicals and improves the function of Adrenal glands. It has anti aging properties; recent research (2009) has indicated that certain compounds found in Astragalus root inhibit genetic degradation as well as having a restorative effect on the Chromosomes *Telomeres.*

- **Panax ginseng:** Possesses Life Extension properties; stimulates the Immune system; Inhibits many types of Cancer and minimizes the toxic effects of Radiation Therapy.

- **Tienchi ginseng:** Adaptogen; it scavenges Hydroxyl Free Radicals and increases stamina in persons who undertake endurance exercises.

- **Chinese yam:** Anti-aging. A tonic and restorative herb – used to enhance vigour. Restore impaired immunological functions.

- **Codonopsis root** *(Dang shen)* - **Key Actions:** Adaptogen, Nervine, Galactagogue, Hypotensive, Digestive, Tonic, Anti-ulcer, Blood tonic, Immune system stimulant Cardiotonic Increases Stamina and Alertness rejuvenating the body.

- **Goji berry** *(Lycium barbarum)*: In Tibet Lycium is known as "longevity fruit" and it is one of the richest sources of antioxidants and other essential nutrients. Make sure that it is cold pressed and not reconstituted.

- **Gorgon fruit:** Anti-aging; Improves sexual ability and energy level in the elderly,

- **Gotu Kola leaf** - Gotu Kola is an Adaptogen and has remarkable rejuvenating properties similar to those of Fo-Ti and Ginseng.

- **Guarana:** Combats the symptoms of premature aging.

- **Fo-Ti** *(He Shou Wu):* is considered an adaptogenic and longevity herb.

- **Maca** *(Peruvian Ginseng)* **- Key Actions:** Adaptogen, Anti-aging, Anti-depressant, Tonic (tones, balances, strengthens overall body functions), Nutritive, Fertility enhancer, Aphrodisiac, Endocrine function support and Anti-fatigue.

- **Noni fruit:** It has potent anti-aging properties. Noni fruit contains antioxidants and anti-inflammatory properties that can prevent cancer and other medical conditions. Noni fruit antioxidants prevent the oxidation of fats in the blood, which reduces the risk of Heart attacks, Stroke and Arteriosclerosis. Noni fruit can stabilize the blood sugar and insulin; it can be helpful in pre-diabetes and also with Diabetes.

- **Pomegranate (seeds, rind, hulk and white pith):** Contains high levels of potent Antioxidants, which are the body's front line defence mechanism against premature aging and chronic disease, by preventing and repairing the effects of free radical damage to the cells. Pomegranate helps to prevent *liver spots* (lipofuscin), boosts the Immune System and helps to prevent and treat diseases such as Osteoarthritis and Rheumatoid Arthritis.

- **Privet berry:** Used in China to retard the aging process, ailments of the heart and Enhance function of the immune system.

- **Sweet cherry and Sour cherry:** Slows down the aging process. Improve memory, concentration and vision.

- **Tulsi** *(Sacred Basil)***:** It calms the mind. It protects against and reduces the effect of stress.

- **Turmeric:** It scavenges errand free radicals and slows down the neurological aging process. It is also a powerful anti-inflammatory agent.

- **Mangosteen:** is a tropical fruit native to South East Asia. Most of its health benefits are attributable to its rind due to its high content of Xanthones and not the flesh. Mangosteen also contains Catechins and Proantocyanidins, which together with the Xanthones protect the body from the harmful effects of free radicals and oxidative damage; they also reduce the effect of aging and promote health. It may scavenge Hydroxyl Free Radicals and prevent and treat breast, colon, liver cancer and leukaemia.

- **Sea Buckthorn:** An orange colour berry that has been used medicinally in Asia and Europe for hundreds of years. It has bioactive substances and proteins that all play a role in healing and rejuvenation. The flavonoids in sea buckthorn can help cancer patients to recover more rapidly from the effects of radiation and chemotherapy treatment. Clinical trials have shown that sea buckthorn can help normalize liver enzymes and immune system markers in those with inflammation or cirrhosis of the liver, and may help prevent the harmful effects of many toxic substances. This fruit also improves the health of the intestinal mucosa

- **Triphala:** An Ayurvedic herbal combination for rejuvenation and help maintain longevity by rejuvenating bodily cells and tissue. It consists of these three herbs: Amla *(Emlica officinalis)*, Harada *(Terminalia chebula)* and Bihari *(Teminalia bellerica).*

∗∗∗

5. HERBAL FORMULAE[11]

* Energy, Stamina & Longevity

Indications: Low energy, lack of Stamina, Fatigue, Pain and Stress, Adrenal Exhaustion.

Remedies Selected:
- *Fo-Ti*
- *Chinese Date Seed*
- *Ginger*
- *Gorgon fruit*
- *Noni fruit*
- *Suma*

* Life Extension Herbs

Indications: Premature Aging, Low Energy Level, Chronic disease, Adrenal Exhaustion, Poor Libido and Low Immunity.

Remedies Selected:
- *Astragalus Root*
- *Panax Ginseng*
- *Grape Seeds and Grape skins powder*
- *Green tea*
- *Terminalia chebula*
- *Amla*
- *Silica*
- *Goji Berry*
- *Privet Berry*
- *Rhodiola Rosea*
- *Withania (Ashwagandha)*
- *MSM (Dimethyl- sulfonyl-methane)*
- *Vitamin C with Bioflavonoids*

---

[11] These and other appropriate potent herbal combinations may be offered to the patient following a professional consultation and naturopathic appraisal.

* Vigour and Zest

Indications: Adaptogen Tonic, Anti-cancer, Stress and Memory loss.

Remedies Selected:
- *Ashwagandha*
- *Tulsi*
- *Satavari*
- *Amla*
- *Mint*
- *Zest (Citrus rind)*

* Vigour SOD & Catalase Herbs

Superoxide Dismutase (SOD) is an endogenous enzyme, antioxidant and anti-inflammatory agent with anti-aging and cancer preventative properties.

Indications: Chronic Inflammation, Crohn's Disease, Inflammatory Bowel Disease, Corneal ulcers, Burns and Injuries, Exposure to smoke and Radiation[12], Cancer, Liver disease, Heart weakness, Arthritis and Prostate problems.

Remedies Selected:
- *Ashwagandha*   *Green Tea*
- *Brahmi*   *Parsley*
- *Ginkgo biloba*   *Milk Thistle*
- *Amla (Indian Gooseberry)*   *Korean Ginseng*

---

[12] **Exposure to radiation** causes a cascade of free radicals that wreak havoc on the body. Radiation also decimates the body's supply of glutathione, which allows free radicals to run rampant through our body's tissues and organs. Though there might be some kind of hormesis effect with an up-tick of glutathione body defences, it is vital to understand that glutathione levels cannot be sustained without all the precursors being supplied—namely selenium, magnesium and sulphur.

Module 4
CLEANSING & ELIMINATION

Eliminating Toxins Detrimental fungi and Parasites

1. CLEANSING THE BODY

Herbalism is the oldest known form of healing the sick of the world.
Every substance contained in a plant has purpose and significance. These substances that make up the plant complement each other and act as a whole.

The accumulation of toxic waste products in the body is symbolic of a cluttered mind, which leads to fatigue and sickness. Medicinal plants are important elements of traditional medicine in virtually all cultures to help cleanse and restore the individual at the level of form – the effect, **by restoring or enhancing cellular communication**.

The herbal remedies can be used to assist the body in assimilating essential nutrients and eliminating toxic waste matter, be they irritating chemicals, mucous, plaque, by products of metabolism, anaerobic cells and dead cells, or detrimental organisms and their secretions. As we age the body's ability to eliminate waste products diminishes, hence especially at these times it is important that we support the body in the elimination process in order to prevent pain and suffering.

Where the patient is extremely toxic, such as when pharmaceutical drugs have been taken for some time caution is advised. The internal bath[13] to cleanse the bowels will reduce the severity of the detoxification symptoms.

---

[13] Internal bath refers to means of cleansing the colon either by enemas or colonics; however, these may not be suitable for people who have undergone a colorectal surgical procedure.

2. ACID WASTE BUILD-UP

In Naturopathic Principles, it is stated that disease and premature aging result from an excessive accumulation of acidic waste products in the body. These waste products are disposed in various organs via the bloodstream and also the lymphatic system. Sometimes these wastes are left on the walls of the arteries, and over the years spread throughout the body. Alkaline water and alkaline forming foods are advocated. Acid forming foods such as meat and potatoes, fried foods, soft drinks, sucrose and other sugars build up acidic waste products in the body. Besides bad diet, both mental and physical stress can also form acidic deposits in the body.

3. THE YEAST CONNECTION

It shall be noted that not all Yeasts (or Moulds) are detrimental to health; indeed there are some that are very beneficial. Examples of beneficial (Non Toxic) yeasts are *Brewer's yeast, Torula Yeast and Chinese Caterpillar Fungus.*

Detrimental Fungi (such as Candida Albicans in its mutated form) can cause allergies and may be responsible for infections such as Tinea and many other ailments including, headaches, depression, lack of vitality and digestive problems. These organisms are nourished largely by sugars.

People with cancer, leukaemia or tumours are likely to be infested with harmful yeasts such as Candida albicans, parasites and aflatoxins. Some doctors are aware that fungi are a major cause of diseases such as leukaemia and that cancer is a chronic, infectious, fungus disease. Researchers have found fungal spores in every sample of cancer tissue that they studied.

Pharmaceutical antibiotics destroy the normal protective gut bacteria, allowing harmful intestinal yeast and fungi to grow unchecked.

Anti-Fungal, Parasites and Mould Elimination Herbs

These are an important consideration since harmful yeasts, moulds and parasites could be undermining your immune system. These yeasts interfere with Glutamine metabolism and Iron absorption impeding the proper oxygenation of the body, since Iron is one of the most important oxygen supports in the blood – making you feel tired and uncomfortable.

You can perform a simple test if your body is infected with Candida Albicans:

First thing in the morning, **before you put anything in your mouth**, get a clear glass of water, and then work up a bit of saliva and spit it into the glass.

If you have a Candida infection then strings will appear down from the saliva travelling down the saliva, through the water, towards the bottom of the glass or cloudy saliva will sink to the bottom of the glass. If nothing develops in 30 to 45 minutes, you are probably Candida free.

4. PARASITES ELIMINATION

Parasites may be transmitted to humans through insect bites, drinking contaminated water, and eating undercooked meat and fish. Raw fruits and vegetables can harbour parasites. Parasites can get into the body by putting unwashed hands into the mouth after they have been in contact with something that contains parasites. Close contact with companion pets and other animals is another way of acquiring parasites. **The size of parasites can range from microscopic amoebas to worms that can grow a metre or more in length.**

About a third of parasites in humans live in the digestive tract but the same parasites can travel anywhere else in the body. Parasites may be involved in Crohn's disease, ulcerative colitis, arthritis and cancer. So many people that suffer from diarrhoea, gas, constipation, bloating or other digestive problems, as well as skin rashes, fatigue and other symptoms are likely to be affected by parasites. Normally regular bowel movements will eliminate parasites from the system, however, when there is constipation and the residue of the food eaten is not eliminated within about 36 hours then parasites will readily multiply.

5. HERBAL REMEDIES[14]

* Anti-Fungal Herbs
Detrimental Fungi (such as Candida Albicans in its mutated form) can cause allergies and may be responsible for infections such as Tinea and many other ailments including, headaches, depression, lack of vitality and digestive problems. These organisms are nourished largely by sugars.

Cancer Patients practically always show signs of heavy parasitic infestation, as well as the open ileo-caecal valve syndrome.

Indications: Candida Albicans overload and detrimental Yeast Infections, Mould elimination, Bloating, Joints Pain, Low Energy level, Thrush, Tinea.

Remedies selected:
- *Cinnamon*
- *Garlic*
- *Horsetail*

---

[14] These herbal combinations are available at the Bio Natural Research Clinic and they may be offered to the patient following a naturopathic appraisal.

- *Horseradish*
- *Myrrh.*
- *Neem leaf*
- *Nigella Sativa seeds*
- *Pau D'Arco*
- *Mountain pepper (Tasmannia lanceolata)*
- *Vitamin C (ascorbic acid)*
- *Zinc oxide*

NOTE: When the Candida organisms die, yeast toxins are rapidly released into the blood stream, usually in excess of the liver's capacity. A "die off" reaction is felt, where there is a transient worsening of symptoms. Herbs that support liver and kidney function will reduce this tendency.

* Anti-Radiation Formula

Indications: Radioactivity exposure, Inflammations, Cancer.

Remedies Selected:
- *Aloe Vera*
- *Chaparral*
- *Ginkgo biloba*
- *Green tea*
- *Korean ginseng*
- *Kelp*
- *Parsley*
- *Sarsaparilla*
- *Tulsi*
- *Vitamin C*
- *Spirulina*
- *Chlorella*

* Cleansing Herbs

Indications: Toxic overload, Constipation, Digestive Problems, Flatulence, Bad Breath, Chronic Skin Problems.

Remedies Selected:

Bay leaf	Ginger
Cayenne	Neem leaf
Cloves	Peppermint
Cinnamon	Pau D'Arco
Cumin	Slippery Elm
Coriander	Senna
Fennel	Turmeric
Fenugreek	Wormwood
Garlic	Calcium Ascorbate
Ganthoda	

* Liver & Kidneys Herbs

Indications: Liver and Kidney ailments, Inflammations, Alternating Chills and Fevers, Irregular menstruation, Uterine Cramping and Fatigue

Remedies Selected:

▪ Andrographis	Citric acid
▪ Barberry	Cumin seeds
▪ Black walnut green hull	Horsetail
▪ Buplerum	Nettle
▪ Celandine	St John's Wort
▪ Rosemary	Uva-ursi
▪ Schizandra	Gum Acacia
▪ St Mary's thistle	Knotgrass
▪ Hydrangea root	Bicarbonate of Soda

* Lymphatic System Herbs

Indications: Lymphatic congestion, Glandular Swelling.

Remedies Selected:
- *Burdock root*
- *Fenugreek seeds*
- *Calendula flowers*
- *Poke root*
- *Sarsaparilla*

* Parasites Elimination Herbs

Indications: Parasites may be transmitted to humans through insect bites, drinking contaminated water, and eating undercooked meat and fish. Raw fruits and vegetables can harbour parasites. Parasites can get into the body by putting unwashed hands into the mouth after they have been in contact with something that contains parasites. Close contact with companion pets and other animals is another way of acquiring parasites. The size of parasites can range from microscopic amoebas to worms that can grow a metre or more in length.

Remedies Selected:
- *Barberry*
- *Black walnut green hull*
- *Bistort root*
- *Cloves*
- *Garlic*
- *White horehound*
- *Neem leaf*
- *Wormwood*
- *MSM*
- *Ascorbic acid*

* Mould Elimination Herbs

Indications: Parasites, Detrimental yeasts and Mould infestation, Flatulence and intestinal cramps.

Remedies Selected:
- *Cassia Cinnamon*
- *Coriander*
- *Citrus rind*
- *Cumin*
- *Black cumin*
- *Nigella*
- *Nutmeg*
- *Peppermint*
- *Star anise*
- *Schizandra*
- *Ascorbic acid*

* Systemic Cleanser

Indications: Toxic body conditions, Tumours and growths, Digestive problems, Infections and Cancer Prevention.

Remedies Selected:
- *Ajwain seeds*
- *Cat's Claw*
- *MSM*
- *Bloodroot*
- *Calcium Ascorbate*
- *Mint*
- *Ganthoda root (Indian Valerian)*

Module 5
INFLAMMATION

Eliminating the Cause of Inflammation

1. CAUSES OF INFLAMMATION

The inflammatory response is a process by which the body indicates that there are irritants that necessitate elimination. The inflammation itself is a natural response by the body to overcome and heal disease, however, the cause of the inflammation must be gently removed in order for the body to be restored and prevented from becoming seriously diseased. It has been proposed that 80% of inflammations are caused by unhealthy lifestyle.

There are many factors that may initiate an inflammatory response:
- A diet high in meat, salt, coffee and other acid forming foods.
- Tobacco smoking.
- Trans-Fatty Acids.
- Dehydration.
- Infection by Parasites, Detrimental Fungi and Viruses.
- Radioactivity, Radiation therapy.
- Free Radicals Toxic Overload.
- Pharmaceutical drugs such as Glucocorticoids.
- Fluoride (sodium fluoride and silicofluorides).
- Over excitement and grief.

The symptoms of Inflammation are redness, pain and swelling. Acute inflammation is the initial response of injury to tissue. An Immune Response to Antigens released during the acute or chronic stages of the inflammatory process.

Antigens are molecules or particles of matter that the body regards as foreign or dangerous. For example Cancer cells and detrimental micro-organisms are treated as Antigens by the Immune System. The body in response and to counteract Antigens produces antibodies.

Pharmaceutical Glucocorticoids[15] may allow Antigens to proliferate.

The chronic stage of inflammation generally occurs following the suppression of the inflammatory symptoms by inappropriate medical procedures that focus primarily on treating the symptoms whilst neglecting to adequately consider the causes that initiate the inflammatory process.

2. INFLAMMATION AND DISEASE

It has been proposed that inflammation plays a major role in the Aging Process and is the Root-Cause of many modern diseases. The "free-radicals" generated by the inflammatory process can attack virtually every tissue of the body in a domino-like cascade. Such tissues include Brain (depression and dementia), Blood Vessels (hypertension and cardiovascular disease), Endocrine Glands (thyroid disease, diabetes), Skin (psoriasis, rosacea, acne, dermatitis, ulcers, hives etc.), and Bone (osteoporosis, arthritis) to name just a few.

Chronic inflammation is an indication that something is wrong in the body, manifesting as various forms of sickness such as: atherosclerosis, cancer, heart valve dysfunction, obesity, diabetes, congestive heart failure, digestive system diseases, Skin Disease and Alzheimer's disease (Brouqui et al. 1994; Devaux et al.

---

[15] Glucocorticoids are a group of Corticosteroid Hormones synthesized by the Adrena Glands in response to Stress. Excessive Glucocorticoids production may suppress various aspects of the Immune System and may cause the destruction (Catabolism) of Connective Tissue.

1997; De Keyser et al. 1998). In aged people with multiple degenerative diseases, the inflammatory marker, C-reactive protein, is often sharply elevated, indicating the presence of an underlying inflammatory disorder (Invitti 2002; Lee et al. 2002; Santoro et al. 2002; Sitzer et al. 2002). When a cytokine blood profile is conducted on people in a weakened condition, an excess level of one or more of the inflammatory cytokines, e.g., TNF-a, IL-6, IL-1 (b), or IL-8, is usually found (Santoro et al. 2002).

3. FOODS THAT CAUSE INFLAMMATION

Inflammation in the body can be mediated by dietary considerations, by avoiding those foods that are inflammatory, listed below, and consuming foods that do not cause inflammation (anti-inflammatory foods).

- Refined sugars, sucrose, corn syrup, and artificial sweeteners.
- Excessive use of refined carbohydrates.
- Pasteurised & homogenized cows milk, Ice cream, Cheddar cheese.
- Margarine.
- Unfermented soy products e.g. Soymilk and Soy oil.
- Seafoods that are garbage eaters such as Oysters.
- Genetically modified food (GMO) – at present about 50% of Soy and Corn is genetically modified.
- Processed foods, fast foods, canned foods, deep-fried foods.
- Microwave-cooked/heated foods.
- Potato chips or French fries, pretzels.
- White bread, white flour white pasta, white rice and starches generally.
- Preserved meats, smoked meats and smallgoods (bacon, ham, hot dogs, salami sausages).
- Commercially prepared Snack foods.

- Hydrogenated vegetable oils/oils that are not cold pressed: (canola, cottonseed oil, olestra, regular peanut, safflower, corn, sunflower, cotton seed and mixed vegetable oils).
- Soft drinks, soda and manufactured caffeinated drinks.
- Canned, bottled or frozen fruit juices.
- All teas in tea bags. Black tea.
- Coffee excessive use.
- Peanuts, peanut butter excessive use (due to contamination by mould Aflatoxins).
- Overcooked foods; left over foods and fried foods.
- Commercial table salt (the body recognises this chemically treated sodium chloride as corrosive poison to its cells. This causes constant overburden for our excretive organs. Common table salt also has toxic additives like anti-caking agents (Sodium silico-aluminate), flowing agents (tricalcium phosphate) and preservatives, which are not listed on the label). We need whole natural mineral salt in our diet – Celtic sea salt, Himalayan salt and Indian black salt (Kala Namak) are recommended and they contain minerals and trace elements that are essential to the body.

4. ANTI-INFLAMMATORY FOODS

- **Deep sea Fish** (wild salmon, sardines, tuna, herrings, snapper, cod, rainbow trout, whitefish, halibut).

- **Fresh whole fruits** (avocados, apples, blueberries, fresh pineapple, kiwifruit, lemons, limes, papaya, raspberries, strawberries). Honeydew melon and cantaloupe are generally not recommended).

- **Vegetables** (asparagus, bell peppers, bok choy, broccoli, Brussels sprouts, cabbage, cauliflower, chard, collards, fennel bulb, garlic, green beans, green onions, spring onions, kale, leeks, olives, spinach, sweet potato, turnip greens. Avoid the nightshade family of plants such as potato, tomato and eggplant, as these may actually make the pain from inflammation worse).

- **Omega-3 essential fatty acids** are very powerful anti-inflammatory agents. Fish Oil, Chia seeds and Flaxseeds are an excellent source of Omega-3.

- **Evening primrose oil:** Known to suppress inflammations, and it is also useful in the treatment of Acne, Eczema, Chronic Fatigue Syndrome, Fibrocystic Breast Disease and Scleroderma.

- **Soybean products** that are fermented and non-genetically modified may help reduce pain and inflammation.

- **Cold pressed Extra virgin olive oil, hemp seed oil and flaxseed oil, avocado oil, coconut oil** (it is better not to heat these oils).

- **Nuts, legumes and seeds** (almonds, flaxseed, hazelnuts, sunflower seeds and walnuts, which are high in antioxidants and vitamin E).

- **Dark green leafy vegetables** (beware of pre-packed mixed salad sold in cellophane or plastic bags, which is treated with chlorine).

- **Aloe Vera –** juice consumed orally contains the enzyme *Bradykinase* that may reduce inflammation that occurs within the digestive tract. Excellent remedy for skin inflammation.

- **Spirulina and Chlorella**: these blue-green algae are antioxidant and nutrient rich Tonic-Super-Foods that are anti-inflammatory, cleansing and immunity enhancers. Both of these nutrients would benefit people who suffer from various medical conditions. Supplementation with both of these algae has been looked to as possible method of mitigating exposure to heavy metals.

- **Barley grass -** it facilitates the healing of the colon tissue and minimizes inflammation by reducing the Tumour Necrosis Factor-alpha (TNF-a).

- **Deer velvet antler:** It has Anti-Cancer and Anti-Inflammatory properties; it improves Immune System. The Anabolic or growth promoting effects of Velvet Antler have been well documented.

- **Propolis:** In 1987 Oxford University found that Propolis contained 149 active substances with strong anti-oxidant and anti-aging properties.

- **Reishi mushrooms:** Adaptogen; Stimulates Immune Function; Inhibits Inflammation and diminish the sensation of Pain.

- **Sea cucumber:** known to alleviate inflammation associated with Painful Joints, Damaged Ligaments, Tendonitis, Sprains and Rheumatoid Arthritis.

- **Bromelain** (derived from pineapple): is a group of closely related compounds consisting of

Proteolytic and other Enzymes. Bromelain has the ability to reduce inflammations in such conditions as: Ulcerative Colitis, Ulcers, Joint Pain, Arthritis, Gout and Burns.

- **Quercetin** food sources: green tea, black tea, organic apples, red onions, fennel leaves, lemon, dill, spring onions, hot green chillies, cranberries, black grapes, hawthorn berries, elderberries, cocoa, lovage and boneset.

- **Black cumin** *(Nigella sativa):* inhibits the release of histamine from mast cells and inhibits the activity of lipoxygenase (lipoxygenase is a group of endogenous Fatty Acid Metabolising Enzymes).

- **Cat's claw:** useful in inflammatory diseases such as Arthritis, Bursitis, Gout, Shingles, Lupus and Inflammatory Bowel Disease.

- **Jojoba oil, neem oil, emu oil, calendula, tea-tree oil** (applied externally).

- **Fruits that are high in antioxidants:** Bilberry, Cherries, Goji berries, Acai berries, Mangosteen, Pomegranate (rind and seeds) and Sea Buckthorn.

- **Diatomaceous Earth (food grade):** also known as *Fossil Shell Flour.* It is a good source of important minerals and trace elements especially *Silica*, which has a direct relationship to mineral absorption. *Silica fades age spots* and stimulates metabolism for higher energy levels. *Silica* works with other Antioxidants to prevent *premature aging.*

- **Liquorice root extract:** this is a systemic anti-inflammatory herb that also restores the Adrenal Glands.

5. HERBAL REMEDIES

* Anti-Inflammatory Formula

Indications: Inflammatory diseases, Rheumatoid Arthritis, Osteo-Arthritis, Inflammatory Bowel Disease, Bursitis, Irritable Bowels Syndrome, Crohn's Disease and Ulcerative Colitis.

Selected Remedies:
- *Baical skullcap*
- *Boswellia serrata*
- *Buplerum*
- *Curcumin*
- *Turmeric*
- *Ginger*
- *Piperine*

* Green Super-Foods Combination.

Indications: Exposure to Radioactivity. Inflammations, Colitis, Arthritis, Cancer, Low Immunity and Toxic Overload.

Remedies Selected:
- *Spirulina*
- *Chlorella*
- *Barley grass*
- *Moringa oleifera*
- *Ginger*

* Joints & Muscle Formula

Indications: Joints pain and Inflammation, Muscle and tendons pain and Inflammation, Fibromyalgia.

Remedies Selected:
- *Boswellia serrata*
- *Curcumin*
- *Piperine*
- *Glucosamine*
- *Celery seeds*
- *Bovine collagen*
- *MSM*
- *Vitamin C*

* Super Herbal Antioxidants

Indications: Stress, Chronic Diseases, Chronic Fatigue Syndrome, Premature Aging, Weakness and Free Radicals toxic overload.

Remedies Selected:
- *Ashwagandha,*
- *Grape seeds powder*
- *Grape skin powder*
- *Green tea*
- *Cacao (raw unprocessed)*
- *Acai berry*
- *Fo-Ti*
- *Reishi mushrooms*

NOTE
The above Herbal Combinations and other remedies are available through the Bio Natural Research Clinic at Dandenong South (see page 100), and may be offered to the patient following a professional Naturopathic Appraisal.

Module 6
HERBAL WISDOM
Powerful Natural Herbal Remedies

Foods and Herbs that heal and revive

Foods and Herbs that Heal and Revive

Herbs can provide the body with the vital elements for nourishment and cleansing. It is wise to become acquainted with the various beneficial herbs that nature provides and how they could benefit you, especially in times of undue stress, sickness and lowered vitality. It appears that for every ailment that afflicts humanity and other creatures there is a remedy provided by Nature, but you need to know what is required and what is appropriate for you. Animals have their instinct regarding their herbal medicinal needs; humans seem to have lost their intuitive intelligence as they depend more and more on technology and man-made chemicals for diagnosis and treatment.

There is a natural drug-free solution for any physical and mental problem. You need to make the effort to be better informed.

1. Revitalize with Water and Lemon Juice

This is a simple solution when you feel overly tired especially after a large meal. It is likely to be because your body is not getting enough water. Simply have about 300 ml glass of purified water with the juice of one lemon and drink it slowly. It should increase your level of vitality within minutes!

2. How to Stop Gastric Reflux

Have an apple at night before retiring. Then use the Digestive Tonic (refer to page 72)

3. Castor Oil for healthy skin

Castor oil has many medicinal and curative uses when applied externally. The Rinoleic Acid in castor oil inhibits many viruses and bacteria and as castor oil is able to penetrate skin tissue deeply, this makes it an effective treatment for Acne.

Castor oil packs have been used for dissolving tumours, moles and warts, and to improve circulation and elimination.

Castor oil packs (4 minutes hot and 1 minute cold) have been used to bring relief from painful liver congestion.

Castor oil, when massaged into Hair, reputedly promotes Hair Growth and it also alleviates Rheumatic or Arthritic pain.

4. Burns Treatment with Egg White
Keep in mind this treatment of burns, which is included in teaching beginner fireman this method. First aid consists to spraying cold water on the affected area until the heat is reduced and stops burning the layers of skin. Then, spread egg whites on the affected area.

5. Cinnamon and Honey
Mix one tablespoon of raw honey wit half teaspoon of powdered cinnamon, for Cold & Flu, Chronic Coughs and Sinusitis.

6. Selected 14 Herbs Main Uses
The following list of herbs is that can be useful to alleviate disease and suffering. There are many other herbs that nature provides for the benefit of humankind and animals but one needs to be informed about what's available in nature. In my book "The Revival of Herbal Wisdom" some of this knowledge is offered for the enquiring and open minded.

(i) Albizia *(Albizia lebbeck)*

Albizia binds digested food and helps the intestines to absorb water. It is used in Ayurvedic medicine for Asthma and Eczema. It is useful for the treatment of diarrhoea, Asthma, Bronchitis, Hayfever and Eczema.

(ii) Arjun *(Terminalia arjuna)*

Arjun is a potent and effective Ayurvedic herb used to treat many heart conditions. It is useful in the treatment of Angina, Hypertension, Tachycardia and coronary artery disease.

(iii) Bistort *(Polygonium bistorta)*

The roots of this medicinal plant are edible, either raw or fire roasted, having similar flavour to chestnuts. Bistort has many medicinal uses such as: Malaria, Irritable Bowels Syndrome, Diverticulitis, Stomach Ulcers and to improve Blood Circulation.

(iv) Black Cohosh *(Actaea racemosa)*

Native Americans have used this herb for the relief of the symptoms of Menopause such as Hot Flushes and Mood Swings. It is a useful remedy for sedating the Nervous System, Whooping Cough, Uterine Fibroids and Cysts and Tinnitus.

(v) Dulse *(Rhodimenia palmata, Palmaria palmata)*

Dulse and other sea vegetables such as Kelp and Wakame are a rich source of Iodine, however they must be sourced from unpolluted areas since these sea plants absorb heavy metals and radiation. **Iodine is utilized by every hormone receptor in the body.** The absence of iodine causes a hormonal dysfunction that can be seen with practically every hormone inside the body. It has been shown that patients with insulin resistant diabetes have a partial to full remission of their illness in the presence of taking iodine. Iodine deficiency is also felt to be the source of ovarian cysts. With iodine replacement therapy the cysts disappear and women have stopped having **ovarian cysts**.

Did you know that 1 in 3 humans are iodine deficient? According to WHO, in 2007, nearly 2 billion individuals had insufficient iodine intake, a third being of school age.
Iodine deficiency can have serious consequences, causing abnormal neuronal development, mental retardation, congenital abnormalities, spontaneous abortion and miscarriage, congenital hypothyroidism, and infertility.
 Later in life, intellectual impairment reduces employment prospects and productivity. Thus iodine deficiency, as the single greatest preventable cause of mental retardation, is an important public-health problem.

(vi) Moringa *(Moringa olifera)*
This fast growing tree originated in Northern India and is used to prevent and treat over 300 diseases - an impressive range of medicinal uses with high nutritional value. Moringa is considered one of the world's most useful trees. The leaves contain complete proteins, which are rare to find in the plant kingdom. It is high in Calcium, Potassium, Vitamins A and C; provides a rich and rare combination of **Zeatin, Quercetin, Beta-sitosterol, Caffeoylquinic acid and Kaempferol.**[16].

Moringa leaf is useful in the treatment and prevention of Cancer and Premature Aging, Malnutrition, Varicose Veins, Diabetes, Hypertension, Liver Disease, and Anaemia. It offers protection against Radiation.

---

[16] Anwar F, Latif S and others, Dept of Chemistry, Univ of Agriculture, Faisalabad-38040 Pakistan.

(vii) Golden Root (*Rhodiola rosea*)
Rhodiola rosea is a potent Anti-Aging herb. It is useful in the treatment of Chronic Stress, Chronic Hepatitis, Fibromyalgia, Headaches and Migraines, Anxiety and Depression, Lungs Inflammation and to boost Energy Level.

(viii) Boswellia *(Boswellia serrata)*
Boswellia is an Indian herb utilized in Ayurvedic medicine.

Researchers have found that this herb blocks a lethal pro-inflammatory enzyme called 5-lipoxygenase, a potent contributor to inflammatory processes involved in many diseases such as cancer, atherosclerosis, arthritis, inflammatory bowel disease and asthma.

Boswellia's many medicinal uses include: Crohn's Disease, Ulcerative Colitis, Psoriasis, Arthritis and Gout, Chronic Pulmonary Disease, Leukaemia and **Brain Cancer.**

(ix) Bugleweed *(Lycopus virginicus)*
This herb is used specifically for Hyperactive Thyroid Gland and Grave's Disease. It is also useful for Coughs, Respiratory Diseases and Sleeplessness.

(x) Cinnamon *(Cinnamomum zeylanicum, Cassia cinnamomum)*
Cinnamon can kill many types of detrimental organisms; it is a powerful natural remedy to eliminate the flu virus. It is the traditional remedy used for nosebleeds. It helps to prevent heart disease and lowers elevated blood sugar level in diabetes.

(xi) Fo-Ti *(Polyganum multiflorum)*
It is considered one of China's four great herbs and is used in an alternating basis with Ginseng. It is considered an adaptogenic and longevity herb and plays an important part in balancing all the body systems, with particular focus on the Immune System.

It can be used to improve memory and mood, mental clarity, concentration, alertness and focus. Used to restore hair growth and colour; for erectile dysfunction; it improves energy and stamina. It has anti-cancer activity – inhibits tumour cells and reduces high blood pressure in Hypertension.

(xii) Liquorice Root *(Glycyrrhyza gabra)*
Liquorice root is a systemic anti-inflammatory. It is useful in cases of peptic ulcers, asthma, bronchial problems and cough. It is especially useful in the treatment of adrenal exhaustion.

(xiii) Nigella *(Nigella sativa)*
This herb is also known as Black Cumin. The seed has been used for centuries to treat respiratory and digestive problems, parasites, and inflammation.

Nigella seeds and oil inhibit the development of **Pancreatic Cancer**. This herb strengthens the Immune System and increases body vigour. It is useful in respiratory illness such as Bronchopneumonia and Asthma. It is also useful in the treatment of Allergies and Skin Conditions such as Eczema, Boils and Psoriasis. It promotes smooth skin and shiny hair. It sharpens eyesight.

(xiv) Wild Yam *(Discorea villosa)*
This herb is primarily used as a visceral relaxant and antispasmodic.

It has many medicinal uses such as to alleviate period pains, Endometriosis, Morning Sickness, Post Natal Depression, Infertility and PMS. It has Anti-aging and anti-cancer properties.

It is used for Hepatitis and Haemorrhoids with pain in the liver, Angina Pectoris and Lower Back Pain and to enhance Libido.

7. Digestive Tonic Herbs

Indications: Gastric reflux (GERD), Esopharyngeal reflux (EPR), Weak digestion.

Contains the following Herbs:
> *Ajwan*
> *Anise*
> *Bistort*
> *Ganthoda root (Indian Valerian)*
> *Ginger*
> *Cardamom*
> *Digestive Enzymes*

NOTE: Tamarind tea and Sumac are used in Ayurvedic medicine for Gastric Reflux.

Module 7

NUTRITIONAL DEFICIENCY SYMPTOMS

Vitamins, Minerals, Enzymes, Amino Acids, Essential Fatty Acids, Fibre and Water

A WORD ABOUT SUPPLEMENTS

There is an axiom that states: "The whole is greater that the sum of its parts" and my experience tells me that this is correct.

Modern man tends to separate, divide and subdivide to analyze things in order to find out what works, however, each perceived separate part is related to other parts and all these perceived separate parts have a co-dependency. Nature tends to combine required nutrients in a synergistic fashion whilst man, under pressure from giving a convenient scientific explanation bound to commercial interests tends to divide and give things a separate identity.

Every nutrient will depend on other nutrients and body conditions for its utilization, when these other needs are not met, the isolated supplement cannot be utilized. For example all anti-oxidant /enzymes depend on the endogenous anti-oxidant enzymes produced by the body (Glutathione peroxidase, Superoxide Dismutase (SOD) and Catalase; the body's production of these powerful anti-oxidants depend on the body's secretion of Redox Signaling molecules. These essential factors have been proven to decrease with the aging process. Glutathione production and activity requires Copper and Selenium, and Iodine is essential for the utilization of Selenium. Natural remedies and nutrients have been discovered to re-establish the production of these essential body secretions so as to protect against illness and premature aging.

Whilst manufacturers recognize the need to combine several different nutrients together, they cannot match Nature's wisdom in combining the supposedly separate parts into a whole. The power of Nature, however, is greatly hampered by man's interference by using chemical fertilizers, hybridizing plants and lately Genetically Modified plants.

There will be spokespersons with credentials to their name that will tell you that GMO food is safe, Micro waved food is safe, Chemical Additives to food and drinks are safe and Pharmaceutical Drugs are scientifically based whilst Natural Medicine is unproven etcetera! To this I will say that, "The truth is not of this world, but it can be heard in this world" so you need to free your mind of rigidly held beliefs that are simply not true. It is good to be informed by sources that are not biased or bound by commercial interests or political pressure.

Where possible, the best way to obtain these essential nutrients is through organically grown or wild-crafted produce. When this is not readily available, when the food you eat is grown on depleted or contaminated soils and its nutritional value is destroyed through processing and cooking; when the water and fluids you drink are contaminated with chemicals then the need for supplements that are natural and not synthetically produced may be of significant benefit.

Last but not least, changes and adjustments in diet and lifestyle should be seriously considered and implemented with the assistance of a caring and competent physician.

***

SYMPTOMS & POSSIBLE DEFICIENCY
Alphabetical listing

Abdominal pain:	Zinc. Vitamins B5 & B6. Calcium.
Acne:	Zinc. Vitamins B5 & B6. Glutathione. Calcium. Potassium.
Aggression:	Calcium. Iron. Magnesium. Selenium.
Alkalosis[17]:	Arginine. Chlorine.
Allergies:	Low HCl[18]. Manganese. EFA[19]. Bioflavonoids. *Dehydration causes an increase in histamines.*
Anaemia:	Iron. Copper. Iodine. Vitamins B12, B5, B6, E. Folic Acid. Lysine. Biotin and Selenium. Low hydrochloric acid secretion.

Can be caused by Radiotherapy or Lead Poisoning.

Anal pruritus or itch:	Zinc. *There could be Pin Worms.*
Aneurism[20]:	Copper.
Anorexia:	Sodium. Biotin. Phosphorus. Zinc. Vitamin B6.
Anxiety:	Calcium. Chromium. Phosphorus. Iron. Potassium. Selenium. Serotonin.
Apathy:	Vitamin B12. Folic Acid. Potassium. Sodium. Phenylalanine. Tyrosine. Dopamine.[21] *Check Dehydration.*

---

[17] **Alkalosis** is a condition where the blood and tissues of the body become exceedingly alkaline.

[18] **HCl** is the chemical symbol for Hydrochloric Acid.

[19] **EFA** denotes Essential Fatty Acids.

[20] **Aneurism** refers to an abnormal enlargement of an artery due to a local weakening of the arterial walls.

[21] **Phenylalanine** is a precursor for the production of **Tyrosine** and **Dopamine** in the body.

Arthritis:	Calcium. Vitamin E. Boron. Vitamin C & Bioflavonoids. Potassium. Lack of Sunlight. Sulphur. Phosphorus. Enzymes. Vitamin A. Vitamin B5. Linoleic Acid (Omega 6).
Asthma:	Magnesium. Manganese. Molybdenum. Vitamin B3. *Possible triggers -->Dehydration. Inorganic Chlorine and certain Food Additives.*
Atherosclerosis[22]:	Choline. Magnesium. Chromium. Glutathione.

Atrophy[23] of Testicles: Arginine. Zinc.
*Note: Cadmium accumulates & causes atrophy of the testicles.
        Excessive alcohol causes shrinkage (atrophy) of the testicles.*

Bad-breath (Halitosis): Low HCl. Zinc. Vitamins B3, B6 and C.
Can be caused by Liver Malfunction.

Belching:	Low HCl.
Bell's palsy:	Calcium. Vitamin B3. Vitamin B12.
Bleeding gums:	Bioflavonoids. Vitamin C.
Bleeding ulcers:	Bioflavonoids.
Bloating:	Low HCl. Vitamin B6. Enzymes.

May be a sign of Gluten or Lactose intolerance.

Bone pain:	Vitamin D. Calcium. Phosphorus. Potassium Iodide.
Body odour:	Zinc. Magnesium. Chlorophyll.

Body odour can be due to metabolic imbalance and the effect of toxic substances stored in the body. Eliminate foods that are high in Choline (eggs, fish, liver and legumes).

Bowed legs:	Vitamin D.

---

[22] **Atherosclerosis** is a thickening of the inner coat of arteries by deposition of cholesterol and other substances.
[23] **Atrophy:** a lessening of size and function by disuse.

Bronchial infections: Vitamin A.

Bruising easily: Vitamin C. Bioflavonoids.

Burning in mouth and throat: Vitamin D.

Bursitis[24]:   Vitamin B12. Vitamin C & Bioflavonoids.
Sulphur. *Can be due to Arthritis.*

Calcification of soft tissue: Magnesium (primarily). Vitamin D.
Unused Calcium can lodge itself anywhere in the body.

Capillary dilation: Iron. *Stress causes capillary dilation.*

Capillary fragility: Bioflavonoids. *Can be due to Diabetes.*

Candida albicans: Low HCl. Zinc. Silica.
Can be caused by excessive use of pharmaceutical antibiotics.

Carpal tunnel syndrome: Vitamins B2 and B6. Manganese.
Can result from excessive fluoride[25] ingestion.

Cataracts: Histidine. Methionine. Inositol.
Phenylalanine. Glutathione.
Allopurinol (drug prescribed for Gout) can cause cataracts.

**"Chicken Skin" on
back of arms:**   Essential fatty acids (EFA).

Chronic liver disease: Choline. Essential Fatty Acids (Omega-3 and
Omega-6). Vitamin B6. Vitamin E.

Chorea[26]:   Choline. Vitamin E.

Cirrhosis[27] (Liver):   Choline. Glutathione. Magnesium. Zinc.
Selenium. Vitamin B6.

---

[24] **Bursitis** refers to inflammation of the outer covering (bursa) of a group of muscles.
[25] **Fluoride:** from drinking water, toothpaste and foods such as soybeans products, which may have been treated with (fumigated) toxic *hydrogen fluoride* gas.
[26] **Chorea** refers to a nervous condition characterised by involuntary movements of limbs and face.

Can be caused by Alcohol.

Coeliac disease[28]:   Copper. Iron. Folic Acid. Vitamin A. Vitamin K. Vitamin B12. Vitamin B6. Vitamin E. Vitamin D.

Cold feet: Vitamin E. Vitamin B3 *(Niacin)*. Iodine.
Underactive Thyroid could be the cause - insufficient Thyroxine.

Conjunctivitis[29]:   Biotin. Vitamin A.
Usually there is a bacterial or viral infection of the eye.

Constipation: Fibre. Chlorine. Calcium. Inositol. B1. B5. B12. Potassium. Low Hydrochloric Acid. Arginine. Iodine.
Constipation can be caused by Dehydration.

Cold sores: Lysine. Zinc. Calcium.

Colitis[30]:   Vitamin B1. Vitamin K. Sodium. Copper.

Cows milk allergy: Lactase enzyme. *Intestinal flora imbalance.*

Cracked lips: Vitamin B2.

Cracked skin, on heels & fingertips: Essential fatty acids (EFA).

Cracks all over tongue: Calcium. B2.

Cracks at corners of mouth: Vitamin B2. Folic Acid.

Cramps: Vitamins B6, C, D and E. Magnesium. Calcium. Iodine.
Could be caused by Dehydration or poor venous circulation.

Craving sweets: Calcium. Chromium.
There could be a yeast infection

---

[27] **Cirrhosis:** wasting away of normal liver tissue and replaced by connective tissue.
[28] **Coeliac Disease** is a condition of the intestines where there is sensitivity to gluten, which prevents proper absorption of nutrients.
[29] **Conjunctivitis:** inflammation of Conjunctiva of the Eye.
[30] **Colitis** is an inflammatory bowel disease.

Crohn's disease[31]: Copper. Glutathione. Pancreatic Enzymes. Selenium. Zinc. Folic Acid. Vitamin B12. Vitamin A. Vitamin D.

Crumbling teeth: Iodine.

Dandruff: Vitamin A. Zinc. Essential fatty acids (EFA). Vitamin B6. PABA[32]. Sulphur.
Can be caused by excessive sugar or starches consumption.

Dark circles under eyes: Iron.
Could also be due to lack of sleep or Adrenals Exhaustion.

Decaying teeth: Calcium. Molybdenum. Vitamin D. Fluorine.

Defective intestinal absorption: Zinc.

Deficient tooth enamel: Threonine *(Amino acid)*. Vitamin A. Boron. Calcium fluoride. Magnesium.

Dementia, forgetfulness, and depression: Vitamin B3, B6. Biotin. Folic Acid. Vitamin B12.

Depleted vitality: Vitamin K. Vitamin B2. *Dehydration.*

Depression: Calcium. Zinc. Vitamin C. Magnesium. Folic acid. Potassium. Biotin. Iodine. Vitamins B1, B2, B3 and B5. Glutathione.

Dermatitis: Low HCl. Vitamins B2, B5, B6, E,
Skin inflammation Glutathione. Biotin. Inositol. Zinc.
and Rash Selenium.

Diabetes: Chromium. Vanadium. Manganese. Copper. Vitamin B6. Amino Acids.
(Pancreatic Fluke likely to be involved).

Diarrhoea: Low HCl. Vitamin K. Iron.

Digestive tract infections: Vitamin A.

---

[31] **Crohn's Disease** is a severe form of Colitis usually affecting the lower part of the small intestine (ileum).
[32] **PABA** - Para Amino Benzoic Acid.

Digestive disorders:	Low HCl. Sodium. Iron. Vitamin B5. Enzymes.
Diverticulitis:	Fibre. Probiotics.
Dilated capillaries - nose and cheeks:	Low HCl.
Dizziness:	Iron. Manganese. Vitamin B12. Sodium.
Double vision:	Vitamin A. Vitamin B12.
Drowsiness:	Boron. Tyrosine.

 Drowsiness can be a symptom of Hypoglycaemia & Adrenal Glands Insufficiency or a side effect of Pharmaceutical Drugs.

Dry mouth:	Vitamin B12. *Side effect of many pharmaceutical drugs.*
Dry skin:	Calcium. Vitamin A. Essential Fatty acids. Vitamin C. Iodine.
Ear Wax deposits: (excessive & hard)	Phosphorus. Essential Fatty Acids. *Excessive cheese consumption may cause excessive earwax secretion.*
Eczema:	Calcium. Potassium. Sulphur. Biotin. Inositol. PABA. Vitamin B6. Glutathione. Delta-6 Desaturase enzyme *(Essential for fatty acids conversion).*
Electrolyte[33] abnormalities:	Chlorine.
Enlarged heart:	Vitamin B1. Selenium.
Excessive sweating:	Vitamin D. Omega-6 Essential Fatty Acids.
Excessive thirst:	Omega-6 Essential fatty acids. Potassium.
Exhaustion (fatigue):	Vitamin C. Iron. Zinc. Vitamins B1, B3, B5, B12. Folic acid. Biotin. Potassium. Amino acids. Essential Fatty Acids (EFA).

---

[33] **Electrolyte** refers to a molecule or particle, which has an electrical charge (either positive or negative).

Phosphorus.
Can be due to Dehydration.

**Extremely nervous
& excitable:**   Calcium. Magnesium. Vitamin
B6. Essential Fatty Acids.

Eyes are dry, inflamed & painful: Vitamin A. Vitamin C.

**Eyes are itchy, burning
and watery:**   Vitamin B2.

Eyes are red (bloodshot): Vitamin C. Bioflavonoids. Vitamin A.
Vitamin K. Lysine.

Eyes cannot tolerate light: Vitamin A.

Eyelids are droopy: Vitamin B1. Kali Phos (tissue salts)

Eye pressure *(Glaucoma)*: Chromium. Vitamins B1 & B6. Zinc.
Lipoic acid. Gamma linolenic acid –
GLA (Omega-6 derivative).

Eye sight disturbances: Alpha-Linolenic Acid (Omega-3)
(Improves retina response to light).

Facial neuralgia: Calcium. Amino acids. Vitamin B1.
Herpes simplex virus could be involved.

Fainting sensation: Iron. B5. B12. Manganese.

Fat deposits in liver: Inositol. Vitamin E. Choline. Carnitine.

Fatigue: HCl, Zn, Mg, B5, B12, Omega 3, Iron

Feeling of lump in throat: Calcium. Sodium.

Fibro cystic breasts: Vitamin E. Iodine. Essential fatty acids.

Flatulence: Low HCl. Enzymes. Sodium. Sulphur.
Probiotics imbalance.

Fluid in lungs: Magnesium.
Can be caused by Gossypol, found in cottonseed oil.

Fluid retention: Magnesium. Potassium. Vitamins B1, B6.

Folic acid. Iodine. Bioflavonoids. Sulphur. Amino Acids.

Air Pollution (Nitrogen Oxide), Kidneys Ailments and lack of movement can be the cause of fluid retention.

Gait disorder: Vitamin E. Manganese.

Gastric ulcer: Zinc. Vitamin B2. Lithium. Calcium.

Gastritis: Magnesium.
Can be caused by Excessive Stress, Aspirin and Fluoride.

Gall bladder disease: Fibre. Vitamin C. Choline.
Cotton Seed Oil is toxic to the Gallbladder.

Gingivitis[34]: Vitamins A and C.
Can be caused by Detrimental Bacteria and Candida Albicans.

Glossitis (tongue diseases): Vitamin B-Complex.

Glucose intolerance: Manganese.

Gums are spongy, bleeding, infected (gingivitis): Vitamins A and C.

Greying hair: Manganese. Copper. Zinc. PABA. Vitamin B5. Folic acid.

Haemorrhoids: Calcium. Bioflavonoids.

Hair loss *(alopecia)*: Inositol. Biotin. Vitamins B2 & B5. Folic acid. Zinc. Cysteine. Lysine. Iron.
Under-active Thyroid could be the cause.

Hair loss after pregnancy: Folic acid. Iron.

Hair is dull and lifeless: Vitamins B2 and B3.

Hair is fine and brittle: Zinc. Omega-3 Essential Fatty Acids.
Can occur due to Hypothyroidism.

---

[34] **Gingivitis:** inflammation of the gums.

Hands are dry, cracked
and ache painfully: Vitamin B6.

Hardening of the arteries: Choline. Chromium. Copper,
(Atherosclerosis)   Glutathione.
  Homogenised milk, excessive meats,   peanut oil & tobacco
  smoking can be the cause.

Headaches: Iron. Vitamins B1, B3, B6 and B12.
 Can be a sign of Dehydration or an allergic reaction.

Headache before menses: Iodine.

Headache from mental strain: Silica.

Headache from bright lights: Silica.

Headaches (frontal):   Sodium.

Hearing loss *(age related)*: Vitamins A and E.

Heart palpitations[35]:   Calcium. Vitamin B1. Choline.

Heart pain: Vitamin B Complex (esp B1 and B12)

Heart beat irregular: Calcium. Potassium.
Avoid excessive caffeine.

Heart problems: Folic acid. Biotin. Fibre. Selenium. Carnitine.
                            Choline.

Heart attack: Selenium. Taurine. Magnesium. Carnitine.

Heart rhythm disturbance: Magnesium.

Heart weakness: Selenium.

Heat exhaustion: Sodium.

---

[35] **Heart palpitations** can be a sign of Thyroid over-activity.

Heavy metals[36] toxicity: Germanium. Amino acids.

Herpes simplex outbreaks: Calcium. Lysine. Lithium. Zinc.

High blood cholesterol: Biotin. Choline. Inositol. Fibre.
Vitamin B6. Chromium.

Hot flushes: Vitamin E.

Hypersensitive to touch: Calcium.

Hypertension: Calcium. Potassium. Chromium. Magnesium. *Can be due to chronic Dehydration.*

Hypoglycaemia[37]:   Amino acids. Chromium.

Hypothyroidism[38]:   Iodine. Selenium.
Can be due to excessive Oestrogen retention and Liver malfunction.

Inability to gain weight: Vitamin A. PABA[39].

Inability to adjust to darkness: Vitamin A.

Inability to quench thirst: Iodine.

Inability to tolerate pain.   Vitamin B1.

Indigestion: Low HCl /Enzymes. Iron. Vitamins B1, B3, B5. Sodium.
Eating complex denatured meals can cause digestive problems.

Infections
***(Ear, sinus, urinary, intestinal)*:** Vitamin A.
Inflammation of tissue: Copper. Zinc.

---

[36] **Heavy Metals** can get into the body from chemically contaminated food and water, drugs, amalgam fillings, cosmetics, cleaners, deodorants and air pollution.
[37] **Hypoglycaemia:** low blood sugar.
[38] **Hypothyroidism** refers to an under active thyroid gland.
[39] Para Amino Benzoic Acid (PABA).

Increased blood-clotting time: Vitamin K.

Infertility - *Female:*   Vitamins B6, B12 and E. PABA. Inositol.
Excessive consumption of MSG and Caffeine.

Infertility - *Male:*   *Amino Acids* - Arginine, Carnitine, Taurine.
Essential Fatty Acids - Omega-3 & Omega-6.
Vitamins - A, C, E, B12, Folic Acid.
Minerals - Chromium, Selenium, Zinc.
Co-Enzyme Q10.

Insomnia: Calcium, Magnesium, Vit B1, B3, B5, B6 &
Folic acid. Biotin. Vitamin D and E. EFA[40].
Amino acids. Glutathione.

Irritability & nervousness: Vitamin B5. Magnesium. Silica. Sodium.
Phosphorus. Vitamin B1. Threonine
(essential amino acid).

Itching around rectum: Low HCl. Zinc.
 Can be caused by Pinworms or Fungal infection

Joints pain: Calcium. Vitamin C. *(See bone pain).*
Sulphur.
Ageing and Dehydration can be the cause of joint pains.

Kidney damage: Vitamin E.
 *Can be a long-term effect of Insulin use, caused by Dehydration and
Heavy Metals (nickel, cadmium, lead & mercury).
Excessive Sorbitol & Creatine Monohydrate.
Carbon Tetrachloride causes kidneys damage.
Many pharmaceutical drugs can cause kidneys damage.*

Kidney problems: Vitamin B1. Choline. Essential Fatty Acids.

Kidney stones: Vitamins A, B5 and B6. Calcium. Amino acids.
 Chronic Dehydration can be the cause of kidney stones.

Late menstruation: Zinc.

---

[40] **EFA** denotes Essential Fatty Acids.

Light-headed and dizzy: Dehydration, effect of certain drugs.

Liver spots: Selenium.

Loss of appetite: Vitamin B5. Biotin.

Loss of hearing/tinnitus: Manganese. Vitamin B12.

Loss of mental energy: Iodine. Vitamin B12.

Loss of muscular control: Vitamin B6.

Loss of mother love: Manganese.

Loss of vision: Vitamin B12. Alpha-Linolenic Acid (LNA)
Excess consumption of MSG can be the cause.

Low blood pressure: Iodine. Chromium. Folic Acid. Vitamins B1
                             and E. Sodium. Potassium. Amino acids.
It could be due to Adrenals exhaustion.

Lower back pain: Calcium.
Dehydration is a likely contributing factor.

Lowered immunity: Essential fatty acids. Vitamin A.

Low metabolism: Vitamin B1. Iodine. Selenium.

Low sperm count: Zinc. Folic Acid. Vitamins B12, C and E.

Lungs degeneration: Choline.

Manic depression: Lithium. Glutathione. Folic Acid
Hypothyroidism may cause Manic Depression.

Memory loss: Vitamins B1, B3, and B12. Boron. Choline.
                             Iodine.

Menstrual cramps: Calcium. Manganese. Magnesium. Vitamin
                             B6. Essential fatty acids.

Mood (emotional) swings: Vitamin B1. Folic acid. Vitamin B12.

Note: Tyramine[41] Allergy can cause Mood Swings.

Mouth Ulcers: Lysine. Iron. Vitamins B1, B6, B12, Folic Acid.

Mucous in throat: Calcium. Vitamin D.

Muscle pain/soreness: Vitamins B5 & E. Biotin. Amino acids. Colloidal minerals. Selenium.

Muscle wasting: Vitamin B1. Essential fatty acids (EPA Omega-3). L-Carnitine. Glutamine. Selenium.

Muscle weakness: Vitamins B1, B5, D and E. Potassium. Phosphorus. Magnesium. Sodium. Amino acids. Iodine.

Nails are brittle: Silica. Calcium. Essential fatty acids. Iodine.

Nails have white spots and split easily: Zinc.

Nails are split, peeling, cracked: Essential fatty acids. Biotin. Vitamin A. Low HCl.

Nails have ridges, easily broken, spoon shaped: Iron.

Nausea: Sodium. Vitamin B6. Digestive enzymes. *Check dehydration.*

Nausea after taking supplements: Low Hydrochloric Acid (HCl).

Nervousness & irritability: Calcium. Vitamin B6.

Nervous seizures: Magnesium. Vitamin B6.

Needles & pins sensation: Potassium.

---

[41] **Tyramine** is found in such foods as cheese, salami, chocolate, wine, nuts, bananas and brewer's yeast.

Neuropathy[42]: Calcium. Silica. Vitamins B1, B6 and Folic Acid.

Numbness & burning in hands and feet: Vitamin B1.

Numbness & cramping in arms and legs: Vitamin B6.

Numbness and tingling in arms and legs. Vitamin B12.

Oedema: Sulphur. Potassium. Magnesium.

Oily skin & hair: Vitamin B2.

Osteoporosis: Boron. Calcium. Manganese. Copper. Magnesium.

Osteomalacia: Phosphorus.

Paleness of skin: Iron. Folic Acid.

Pain in calf of leg: Zinc. Vitamins B1 and B5.

Pain in arms and legs: Vitamins B5, B6 and E. Biotin.

Pain in bust at menstruation: Potassium.

Parched lips: Silica.

Patches of pale skin on cheeks: Essential fatty acids.

Petechial *(brown/red small skin spots):* Vitamin C.

Period pains: Calcium. Magnesium. Manganese. Iodine. Vitamins B6 and E. Essential Fatty Acids.

---

[42] **Neuropathy:** ailments of the Cranial nerves, Peripheral Nervous System or the Autonomic Nervous System, usually causing numbness.

Photo sensitivity: PABA.

Poor appetite: Vitamins B1 and B12.

Poor bone growth: Manganese.

Poor circulation: Folic acid. Vitamin E.

Poor coordination: Boron.

Poor memory: Vitamins B1, B3, B12. Boron. Choline.

Pre-menstrual tension (PMT): Calcium. Magnesium.
Excessive Caffeine can increase risk.
It can be due to Candida Albicans.

Progressive limb deformity: Vitamin D.

Prostate gland problems: Zinc.

Psoriasis: Vitamin A. Zinc. Glutathione. <u>Nickel.</u> Folic
acid. Vitamin B12.
   Tissue Salts: Ferrum Phos & Kali Phos.

Purple & blue spots
under skin (Purpura): Bioflavonoids. Vitamin C and Vitamin K
 Above can be depleted by Alcohol, Olestra and Chemotherapy.

Psychotic excitement: Lithium. Vitamins B3 and B6.

Rapid pulse: Magnesium.

Reddening of hair: Manganese.

Red nose: Sulphur.

Relaxed muscle tone: Iron.

Red, painful tongue: Vitamin B3. Folic acid.

Reproductive system disorder: Vitamin E.

Reproduction failure: PABA.

Restless legs syndrome: Vitamins E, B1, B3 (Niacin), B5.
Folic Acid.
(Zinc Met – homoeopathic remedy)

Retarded growth: Vitamin D. Inositol. Iodine.

Rheumatoid arthritis: Copper. *Chronic dehydration.*

Ringing in the ears *(tinnitus)***:** Manganese. Bioflavonoids.
Vitamin D.
Rough & wrinkled skin: Iodine. Silica.

Run-down feeling: Iron.

Runny nose: Vitamin C.

**Scale eruptions on scalp,
cheeks & skinfolds,
especially infants:**   Biotin.

Scaling of skin around nostrils: Vitamin B12.

Scar tissue: Vitamin E. Vitamin A. Vitamin C.

Scooping nails: Iron.

Sensitivity to insect bites: Vitamin B1.

Sensitivity to noise: Vitamin B1.

Sexual problems: Manganese. Zinc.

Slow heart beat: Calcium.

Skin wrinkled: Copper.

Shortness of breath: Vitamin B1.

**Shortness of breath
 during exercise:**   Iron.

Skin disorders such as: Folic acid.

Pale, washed out skin.
Vitiligo. Acne.

Skin has oily scales, scalp,
eyebrows, nose and
behind ears:　　　　　Vitamin B6.

Skin cracks on fingers:　Zinc. Essential Fatty Acids.

Skin surface has accumulated
hard keratin-like material: Vitamins A, B5, B6. Biotin. Zinc.
(Hyperkeratosis)　　　　Manganese. Essential Fatty Acids.

Sinusitis:　　　*Detrimental fungi are the cause of most cases of*
　Chronic Sinusitis. It can be due to gastric problems.

Slack pyloric valve:　Potassium.

Sleepiness:　　　　Vitamin B6. Tyrosine. Boron.

Slow heart beat (bradycardia):　Calcium. Long term Potassium
　　　　　　　　　　　deficiency.

Slowed growth of
hair & nails:　　　　Manganese.

Sore mouth /tongue,
　inflammation:　　Vitamin B12.

Sore throat:　　　　Vitamin C. Vitamin D.

Spinal curvature:　　Fluorine (Calcium fluoride tissue salt).

Spleen[43] enlargement: Vitamin B12.

Steel-wool like hair:　Copper

Stomach acidity:　　Sodium.

Stomach irritation:　Folic acid.

Stunted growth:　　Inositol. Iodine. Potassium. Zinc.

---

[43] **Spleen:** soft ovoid gland situated to the left of the stomach, which removes worn-out blood cells and other waste matter from the bloodstream.

Sugar craving:	Amino acids. Chromium.
	Check Yeast Infection
Sulphur sensitivity:	Molybdenum.

Sweaty odorous feet: Silica.
Could be a sign of kidney malfunction.

Swelling of ankles:	Magnesium.

Teeth - decay:	Vitamin D. Calcium. Molybdenum. Fluorine.
Crumbling:	Iodine:
Deficient enamel:	Vitamin A. Calcium fluoride. Magnesium. Threonine (amino acid). Boron.

Tenderness of heels:	Vitamin B5.

Tender breasts:	Vitamin E.

Tendency to miscarriage: Iodine.

Tingling in fingers and toes: Iron. Vitamin B1.

Tinnitus[44] & loss of hearing: Manganese. Coenzyme Q10. Vitamin B12.
Could be caused by excessive consumption of dietary fats.

Thickening of wrists: Vitamin D.

Thirst (excessive) & dehydration: Essential fatty acid (omega-6).
Note: Use Evening primrose oil supplement.

Tongue ulceration:	Silica. Vitamin B1.

Thyroid swelling:	Iodine.

Uncontrollable Herpes Simplex[45]:	Lithium.

---

[44] **Tinnitus** is a condition where there is constant ear noises or ringing in the ears.
[45] **Herpes** Simplex is a type of Virus.

**Vaginal lips are hard,
   scaly & rough:**   Vitamin A.

Vaginal infections (chronic):   Iron.

Varicose veins: Bioflavonoids. Calcium Fluoride (tissue salt).

Vertigo: Iron. Magnesium. Manganese. Vitamin B12.

Vitiligo: Folic acid. Vitamin C. Vitamin B12.
Insufficient HCl secretion.

Wake up feeling tired: Zinc.

Wax in ear (excessive): Essential Fatty Acids. Phosphorus.

Weakened eyesight: Fluorine[46].

Weakness: Essential Fatty Acids. Vitamin B1, B2, B5,
Magnesium, Zinc, Silicon, Co-Enzyme Q10,
Vitamin C

Weakness of joints: Vitamin C. Vitamin D and Calcium.
*Note: Aspirin and Non-Steroidal Anti-Inflammatory Drugs may
accelerate the process of Joint destruction by Chondroclasts.*

Weight change not due to diet: Iodine.

Whiteheads: Vitamin B2.

White vaginal discharge: Silica.

White spots on nails: Zinc. Calcium.

White spots on skin: Zinc.

Ref: The Natural Healer's Handbook, by Thomas D'Amico.

---

[46] **Fluorine** as it occurs in nature - preferably obtained from organically
grown produce. Such as: Almonds, asparagus, carrots, tomato, bananas.

NUTRIENTS DEPLETED BY DRUGS

Drug	Nutrients depleted
Alcohol	Vitamins A, B1, B2, Biotin, Choline, Niacin, Folic Acid, B15 (pangamic acid) and Magnesium.
Ammonium Chloride *(Cough syrup)*	Vitamin C.
Amphetamines	Vitamin C. Zinc.
Antacids *(Aluminium hydroxide)*	Vitamins A & D. Vitamins B1, (B12, Phosphates & Iron absorption and Folic Acid.
Antibiotics	Vitamins C, K, B2, B6, B12. Decreases Protein Synthesis.
Anti Inflammatory Drugs:	Vitamin C. Vitamin K. Folic Acid. Iron & Potassium.
Anticoagulants	Vitamin A & K.
Antihistamines	Vitamin C.
Aspirin	Vitamins A, B complex and C. Calcium, Potassium, Glutathione and Tryptophan.
Barbiturates	Vitamins A, B1, B12, C, D and Folic Acid.
Caffeine	B1, Inositol, Biotin, Potassium, Zinc, Tyrosine.

Caffeine can also inhibit calcium and iron ussimilation.

Chemotherapy	Taurine, Folic Acid, Vitamins A, K.

*Depletes immune system. Impairs digestion & assimilation of food.
Can cause Anaemia, Liver damage and Leukaemia.
Note: Radiation therapy, which is often used with Chemotherapy, can
also deplete Taurine and Vitamin C; Radiation therapy can cause*

effects such as Dermatitis, Impotence, Muscle Wasting, Anaemia and Cancer.

Colchicine *(Used to treat Gout)*	Beta Carotene. Vitamin B12. Sodium. Potassium. Protein. Impairs Magnesium & Calcium metabolism.
Dilantin	Folic acid, Vitamin D, Carnitine.
Diuretics	Vitamins B complex, Potassium, Magnesium and Zinc.
Laxatives	Vitamins A, D E, K, Calcium and Phosphates.
Oral contraceptives	Folic acid, Vitamins B2, B6, B12, C and E. Glutathione.
Penicillin	Vitamin B6, niacin, Vitamin K and Folic Acid. *Increases Potassium excretion.*
Prednisolone	Vitamin B6, C, D, Potassium, Zinc and Glutamine.
Stelazine	Vitamin B12.
Tetracyclines	Vitamin K, Calcium, Magnesium, Iron and Zinc.
Tobacco (smoking)	Vitamins A, B1, Biotin, Folic acid, C and E. Calcium, Selenium, Vanadium, Carotenoids, Superoxide Dismutase (SOD).

Tobacco smoking accelerates the Aging Process, cause Mental Decline and can be the cause of many serious diseases and medical conditions.

COURSES AND EVENTS

Be Educated *not* medicated

If you feel that the contents of this booklet is relevant and rings true, you may wish to contact us and pursue the matter further through private and/or group sessions or events to explain and clarify the issues raised in this booklet. In any case we offer you our blessings and wish you happiness on your healing life journey.

You have a choice and the power to choose is a great gift. You can choose what is for the greater good and also in your best interest.

Our mission is to empower people to live free from sickness and pain and express their full innate real and true potential.

We are *not* offering you yet another belief system but training and the sharing of factual, essential and vital information, so that you can avoid confusion and see things as they really are more clearly, and thus be able to choose what is in your best interest.

It has been said that: *"Only you can deprive yourself of anything."*

And

"An untrained divided mind can achieve nothing!" There is much to learn and to unlearn as you quieten your mind, expand your vision and level of awareness!

Thomas D'Amico and associates, in conjunction with the Bio Natural research centre will conduct information and training in recovery, health and longevity. Thomas is a Naturopathic Physician, Holistic Teacher and Natural Medicine Consultant with over 20 years experience. Thomas wishes to share this vital information that could be of great benefit to anyone that would choose to expand his/her awareness of the truth and thus be set free from ignorance, suffering and pain.

Contacts for BioNatural Pty Ltd and Thomas D'Amico:

Address: 2B Kirkham Road, Dandenong South, Victoria, Australia 3175

Phone: 1300 144 023

Email: info@naturalhealingknowledge.com

Web: www.naturalhealingknowledge.com

www.ingramcontent.com/pod-product-compliance
Lightning Source LLC
Chambersburg PA
CBHW071057280326
41928CB00050B/2534